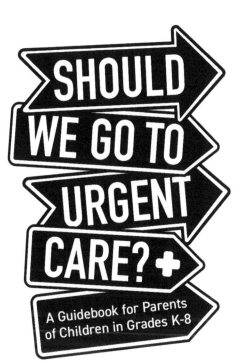

SHOULD WE GO TO URGENT CARE? ✚

A Guidebook for Parents of Children in Grades K-8

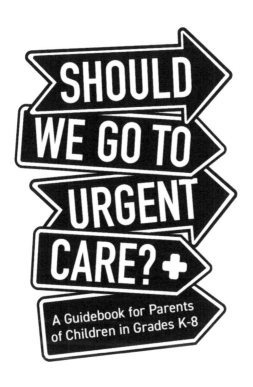

SHOULD
WE GO TO
URGENT
CARE? +

A Guidebook for Parents
of Children in Grades K-8

SARAH IRENE WASHINGTON, MD, FAAP

publish
your gift

SHOULD WE GO TO URGENT CARE?
Copyright © 2021 Sarah Irene Washington
All rights reserved.

Published by Publish Your Gift®
An imprint of Purposely Created Publishing Group, LLC

Printed in the United States of America

ISBN: 978-1-64484-491-5 (print)
ISBN: 978-1-64484-492-2 (ebook)

Special discounts are available on bulk quantity purchases by book clubs, associations, and special interest groups. For details email: sales@publishyourgift.com or call (888) 949-6228.

For information log on to www.PublishYourGift.com

A lot of people resist transition and therefore never allow themselves to enjoy who they are. Embrace the change, no matter what it is; once you do, you can learn about the new world you're in and take advantage of it.

—Nikki Giovanni

*To my daddy, who never got the chance to see
me write my first book.*

*To my mom, who is still here in body,
but your memories are fleeting.*

*You set the example for following The Golden Rule,
being adaptable to change, and continuing to strive
for excellence. I love you both.*

Table of Contents

Acknowledgments

Thank you to Malika for the daily wake up texts and holding me accountable with your check-ins throughout the day. Also thank you to James, Michelle, Doretha, Alexea, Tartania, Dr. Zakiya, Ali, Justine, Una, and all my other family and friends who never stopped believing in me.

Finally, thank you to Dr. Drai for giving me the tools to become a Medical Mogul. This book took way longer than planned and you have been the best business coach guiding me along the way.

Introduction

I excelled academically and musically early in life. I am a classically trained pianist and started playing the piano at the age of 6 or 7. I was an accompanist for my high school choir and occasionally played at church events.

I graduated as the valedictorian of my elementary school. I attended Hampton University as a Presidential Scholar and member of the Honors College, graduating cum laude with Departmental Honors in Biology. I graduated from medical school and completed my Pediatrics residency with a few bumps, but otherwise, it was smooth sailing.

Upon completion of my residency training, I began working at a pediatric urgent care center. Just as I hit my stride as an attending physician, things took a turn. Although I consistently received glowing patient reviews, my employers often criticized the time spent caring for and educating my patients and their families. On March 11, 2018, my father passed away unexpectedly. I became the primary caregiver of my mother, who has Alzheimer's dementia. Once the COVID-19 pandemic hit in March 2020, the company introduced telemedicine quotas and pay cuts. In May 2020, the company relegated me to furlough status after nearly 10 years of employment.

What I initially perceived to be a setback was the perfect setup for a career and lifestyle change, which allowed more time with my mother. I established Kiddo Care Pediatrics to practice medicine on my terms. Now, my patients and parents receive the time and attention they need and deserve. Known for my funny stories, I incorporate humor into my patient interactions, allowing a deeper connection with my patients that builds an even stronger rapport.

When I think about the most asked questions posed by parents, they are by far related to common illnesses and injuries. Parents want to know how these illnesses or injuries occurred, how to treat them, and the timeline for when their child will feel better. Parents often need reassurance that they did the right thing by bringing their child in for evaluation.

Use this book as a textbook for parents who want accurate information from a trusted pediatrician when wondering whether their child may have a particular diagnosis. Each chapter is a clinical vignette that begins with a classic presentation for the listed topic. Next, the diagnosis is provided with general information, common symptoms, and suggested treatment for the given scenario. There is also a section included with injury home care instructions and recommended over-the-counter medications organized in a quick reference list format.

Please note that these are classic presentations and, in life, your child may not always "read the book." There are also atypical presentations of these common illnesses and injuries. If home care is recommended, improvement should be seen within 2-3 days with antibiotic treatment and 3-5 days for viral illnesses. If there is no improvement after that time, you should follow up with your pediatrician. If your child worsens, your child should have a medical evaluation immediately. Finally, this book is a guide. If you have any questions or concerns about your child's condition, you should always contact your pediatrician for medical advice.

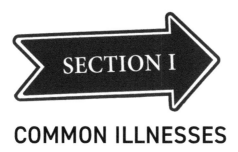

COMMON ILLNESSES

Antibiotic Use

Before we dive into this section on common illnesses, it is important to address appropriate antibiotic use. Most of the illnesses in this book are infectious in origin. A large number of people believe that all infections require antibiotic treatment. This notion is completely false! The reason is that antibiotics only treat bacterial infections. When you take an antibiotic for a viral illness, you take an unnecessary medication. You may be wondering what harm can be caused by taking an antibiotic "just in case." When you take any medication, there is always a possibility of side effects or an allergic reaction. There is no benefit to taking unnecessary medicine. For those whose children fight taking medicine, giving an unnecessary antibiotic is an especially fruitless battle. In addition, taking unnecessary antibiotics can cause antibiotic resistance, which occurs when bacteria no longer respond to antibiotics that previously worked due to antibiotic overuse. As a result, a "stronger" antibiotic with a broader spectrum of bacterial coverage is necessary to treat the infection. These broad-spectrum antibiotics can cause even more side effects. We have guideline criteria for each illness that we use to decide if and when to start antibiotics. You will learn these criteria in their corresponding chapters.

Upper Respiratory Infection (URI/Common Cold)

Sally is a 7-year-old girl who has a 3-day history of cough, runny nose, and congestion. She complains of having an itchy throat but denies having any pain with swallowing. No fever, headache, abdominal pain, vomiting, diarrhea, or rash. She is eating slightly less than usual but is drinking fluids. What does Sally have?

Sally has an upper respiratory infection. Upper respiratory infections (URIs) are infections located in the nose/nostrils, nasal cavity, sinuses, mouth, pharynx (throat), and larynx (voice box). They can cause fever, cough, runny nose, nasal congestion, sore throat, throat itchiness, ear congestion, and ear pain. Most URIs are viral and resolve on their own within 7-10 days. Lower respiratory infections, on the other hand, affect the trachea (windpipe) or lungs.

Treatment is what we call supportive care. Supportive care is treating the symptoms of the illness to make the sick person as comfortable as possible. Tylenol/acetaminophen or Motrin/ibuprofen can be used to treat fever or pain. Staying hydrated is always important. It is more important to drink than to eat. If your child is not eating, this may be the time when you can give more juice than usual since that serves as the primary source of calories. Throat lozenges and saltwater gargles can be used to treat an itchy throat. Nasal saline spray, steamy showers, and a cool-mist humidifier can help with nasal congestion. The primary ingredient in many homeopathic cough syrups like Zarbee's is honey. Honey is soothing for the throat. You can substitute honey in place of the honey-containing homeopathic cough syrups. Limit the honey to 2 to 3 teaspoons per day.

Should Sally go?

No. Uncomplicated URIs resolve on their own in 7-10 days.

Final Care Plan: Sally's parents can practice supportive care and treat her symptoms to keep her comfortable. Remember, it is more important to drink than to eat. Make sure to give your child lots of fluids. Sally's parents should follow up with her pediatrician if there is no improvement in 3-5 days.

Otitis Media (Middle Ear Infection)

Jaden is a 9-year-old boy who started complaining of left ear pain this morning. He has had a runny nose, nasal congestion, and a slight cough for the past 2 days. His highest temp was 100.2°F. No eye discharge or sore throat. He has a normal appetite. What is the diagnosis?

Otitis media is the medical term for a middle ear infection. The middle ear is the region from the tympanic membrane (TM or eardrum) to the Eustachian tube (the inner tube that connects the inner ear to the back of the throat). When people are diagnosed with "ear infections," this is the region of the ear that has been affected. We will talk about outer ear infections a bit later.

How do ear infections occur? Your ears, nose, and throat are all connected in the back of your throat. When a person gets a viral URI, the mucus produced in the nose and throat can flow into the inner tubes of the ears until it reaches the air-filled space behind the tympanic membrane (TM or eardrum). If the fluid sits against the TM too long, the TM can become swollen and infected. This purulent (pus-containing) fluid and bulging of the TM can be seen on exam by using an instrument called an otoscope. Otoscopes have a magnifying glass and light. They can also be used to examine the nose and mouth.

We will only discuss antibiotic treatment criteria for school-age children. Not all ear infections are treated with antibiotics. If a child is above the age of 6 months, antibiotics are started immediately if the patient is diagnosed with a severe infection. This is defined as fluid behind the TM and any of the following:

- A temperature greater than or equal to 102.2°F
- Moderate/severe otalgia (ear pain does not improve with appropriate dosing of over-the-counter pain medications)
- Ear pain for greater than 48 hours at the time of the exam
- Otorrhea (ear drainage) without the diagnosis of otitis externa (OE or swimmer's ear). Otorrhea stemming from a middle ear infection can only occur if there is a perforation (hole or rupture) of the TM, which allows the fluid to drain out of the ear. We will discuss OE diagnosis and treatment later.

If the patient does not meet the criteria for a severe AOM, we use the Watch and Wait method. The Watch and Wait method is appropriate if the patient has mild ear pain (pain improves with over-the-counter pain medications) and a temperature less than 102.2°F for less than 48 hours. If the symptoms resolve during the observation period, the infection was likely viral, and antibiotics would have been unnecessary.

If antibiotics are started, amoxicillin is the treatment of choice because otitis media is caused by *Streptococcus pneumoniae, Haemophilus influenzae* (Hib), *and Moraxella catarrhalis*. The amoxicillin dose is given as a high dose to be the most effective. Amoxicillin is not used if the patient has an allergy or the patient has used amoxicillin within the last 30 days. If amoxicillin cannot be used, Augmentin (amoxicillin + clavulanic acid) or Omnicef (cefdinir) are second-line medications. If those are not viable options, other antibiotics will be started.

Tympanostomy tubes (ear tubes) are small tubes that are surgically placed in the ear tympanic membrane (eardrum) by an otolaryngologist (Ear, Nose, and Throat or ENT) physician. These tubes are also known as myringotomy tubes or Pressure Equalizer (PE) tubes. The tubes are inserted to help fluid drain out of the middle ear to reduce ear infections. Tympanostomy tubes may be offered if your child has 3 ear infections in 6 months or 4 infections in 1 year with 1 episode in the preceding 6 months. If your pediatrician is concerned about these recurrent infections, your child will be referred to a pediatric ENT physician.

Should Jaden go?

No. Jaden meets the criteria for the Watch & Wait method since his ear pain started this morning, his URI symptoms started 2 days ago, and his pain can be managed with over-the-counter pain medications. Antibiotics do not need to be started at this time.

Final Care Plan: Jaden's parents implemented supportive care. His pain was managed with ibuprofen. His symptoms resolved in 48 hours. Jaden should be evaluated if his symptoms do not improve in 2-3 days or immediately if his symptoms worsen.

Conjunctivitis (Pink Eye)

Keith is a 12-year-old boy who woke up with his right eye crusted shut. After opening his eye, Keith's father noticed there was right eye redness and discharge. Keith has been wiping his eye throughout the day, but the discharge keeps returning. The redness did not improve after using an over-the-counter allergy drop. He denies having any eye pain, itchiness, or vision changes. The mother believes that Keith has pink eye. What is the proper term for pink eye?

Conjunctivitis is the medical term for pink eye. It occurs when there is inflammation of the thin transparent layer that covers your sclera (the white part of the eye) and inside the eyelids. Conjunctivitis can be caused by infections, allergies, and chemicals. Infections can be viral or bacterial.

Viral conjunctivitis can accompany a viral upper respiratory infection (URI). Discharge may be seen, but it is usually watery with occasional small amounts of purulent discharge. This form of conjunctivitis resolves on its own without antibiotics.

Bacterial conjunctivitis is diagnosed when a patient has purulent (pus-like) discharge pooling inside the eyelids. The easiest way to distinguish bacterial eye discharge from the discharge seen after awakening (eye crust) is that bacterial discharge continues throughout the day. You can wipe the discharge away only to find that it continues to reappear.

Both viral and bacterial conjunctivitis are extremely contagious. Hands should be washed before and after touching near the eye or giving eye medications to help prevent the spread of the infection. Allergic conjunctivitis is caused by an allergic reaction, which affects the eye. This will be discussed in greater detail in the allergic rhinitis chapter. Chemical conjunctivitis occurs when a substance gets into the eye and may require eyewashes to flush out the eye.

Most bacterial eye infections are treated with antibiotic eye drops or ointment. Examples of antibiotic eye drops are Vigamox (moxifloxacin), Ocuflox (ofloxacin), Tobrex (tobramycin), and Polytrim (polymyxin B sulfate and trimethoprim *ophthalmic* solution). Examples of antibiotic eye ointment are erythromycin and ophthalmic bacitracin. Ophthalmic bacitracin ointment is specially made to be safe for the eye.

Whenever your child is being evaluated for conjunctivitis, the ears should also be examined. When the ears and eyes are infected simultaneously, it is called otitis-conjunctivitis syndrome. Otitis-conjunctivitis syndrome is usually caused by a bacterium classified as nontypeable *H. influenzae* (different from Hib). The antibiotic of choice to treat nontypeable H. flu is oral Augmentin (amoxicillin + clavulanic acid).

*Medication Administration Tip

FOR EYE DROPS – There are two ways to administer eye drops. For both methods, your child must look straight up. This can be accomplished by leaning the head all the way back while sitting or having your child lie flat on his or her back. Method #1: While your child is looking up, pull down on the lower lid to place the drop into the eye. Method #2: Administer the drop while your child's eye is closed. Aim the drop toward the middle corner of the eye. The drop should fall into the eye once the lid opens. You may need to administer 2 drops to ensure that the medication gets into the eye.

FOR EYE OINTMENT – With the head leaning back, pull down the bottom eyelid and apply a ½ inch ribbon of ointment inside the lid. If you cannot place the ointment inside the lid, you can apply the ribbon over the eyeball. When your child blinks, the medication will be inside the lids. Some children may complain of a short period of eye blurriness after applying ointment.

Oral antibiotics are used if symptoms do not resolve after using eye drops or if there is a concurrent infection such as an ear infection.

Should Keith go?

Yes. Keith should have an eye exam along with an ear exam to ensure that he does not have otitis-conjunctivitis syndrome.

Final Care Plan: Keith was afebrile. Upon eye exam, the right eye was red and purulent discharge was seen pooling inside the right lower lid. The ears and throat were normal. Keith was given a course of Ocuflox and his right eye started to improve in 2 days. As instructed, Keith continued the drops for the full week.

Sinusitis (Sinus Infection)

Ashley is a 14-year-old girl who went to her pediatrician after having cough, runny nose, and nasal congestion for 8 days. No ear infection or throat infection was seen. Parents continued to provide supportive care for the past 3 days. Ashley is now complaining of headaches, which started 2 days ago. No fever. She has been using nasal saline spray, over-the-counter cough medicine, and her humidifier. Ashley has had her symptoms for a total of 11 days. Why isn't Ashley feeling better?

Ashley has sinusitis. Sinusitis is inflammation of the sinuses (air-filled cavities inside of the facial bones within the forehead, cheeks, and nose). Your sinuses create a thin layer of mucus, which traps dust, germs, and other particles that enter your nose. This mucus flows to the back of the nose into the throat where it is either spit out or swallowed. If you have a runny nose, that mucus can also flow forward out of your nostrils. When the sinuses become inflamed, mucus gets trapped in the sinuses. This can cause sinus headaches. As with the eyes, sinus inflammation can be caused by allergic triggers, viruses, and bacteria.

In order for a sinus infection to be clinically diagnosed as bacterial in origin, certain criteria need to be met. The patient needs to either have symptoms that last for at least 10 days OR an initial improvement of symptoms with a sudden worsening such as a fever.

When the cause is bacterial, antibiotics are needed. In addition to the bacteria seen in otitis media, Nontypeable *H. influenzae* is one of the main bacteria that causes bacterial sinusitis. Therefore, the drug of choice is high-dose Augmentin (amoxicillin + clavulanic acid). If there is a mild amoxicillin allergy such as a rash, Omnicef (cefdinir) may be used as an alternative. If there is a severe amoxicillin allergy such as anaphylaxis, other medications need to be used. For older teens and adults, Levaquin (levofloxacin) is an option. Of note, Zithromax (azithromycin) is not a good choice for sinusitis.

Should Ashley go?

Yes. At this point, Ashley meets the criteria for the diagnosis of bacterial sinusitis (sinus infection).

Final Care Plan: Ashley has no allergies to any medications, so she was prescribed a 10-day course of high-dose Augmentin. She continued using the OTC medications, nasal spray, and cool mist humidifier. She started having mild improvement in 2 days.

Strep Throat

James is an 8-year-old boy who has had fever, headache, throat pain with swallowing, and abdominal pain for the past 2 days. He vomited once last night. No fever, cough, runny nose, nasal congestion, or ear pain. No diarrhea or rash. What is the diagnosis? Which symptoms make it less likely to be a viral URI?

James has Strep throat. Strep throat is caused by group A Streptococcus (*S. pyogenes*). This is important because there are other streptococcal strains, but they do not cause Strep throat. Common symptoms of Strep throat are sudden onset of sore throat, pain with swallowing, and fever. Other symptoms are headache, abdominal pain, and nausea with or without vomiting. When you look into your child's mouth, you may see a red throat, red spots on the soft palate, and tonsillar exudate (pus on the tonsils). Swollen lymph nodes (glands) can be palpated in the front of the neck. When Strep throat presents with a red, sandpapery rash, the diagnosis is Scarlet fever. Treatment is the same. Cold symptoms such as cough, runny nose, and nasal congestion are not usually seen with Strep throat.

When patients present with symptoms of Strep throat, testing is performed to confirm the diagnosis. Rapid Strep tests are screening tests, which take 5-10 minutes for results. If the test is positive, antibiotics are started. If the test is negative, a throat culture can be sent to a laboratory for confirmatory testing. Throat cultures usually take 2-3 days for final results.

The treatment of choice is amoxicillin. When treating Strep throat, amoxicillin does not need to be prescribed as a high dose. If your child has a mild amoxicillin allergy, a cephalosporin (e.g. Cefdinir/Omnicef) may be used. If the amoxicillin allergy is severe, Zithromax/azithromycin may be used. Of note, when Zithromax is used to treat Strep throat in younger children, the Strep dosing is 5 big doses instead of the big dose and 4 smaller doses for other infections.

Should James go?

Yes. He should have his throat swabbed from Strep prior to starting antibiotics.

Final Care Plan: James tested positive for Strep throat and was prescribed amoxicillin to treat his infection. To treat his throat pain and fever, he continued to use acetaminophen and saltwater gargles. He began to feel better in 1.5 days.

Serous Otitis Media (Ear Effusion/Fluid in the Ear)

Eddie is a 6-year-old boy who presents with a 3-day history of left ear pain and difficulty hearing out of that ear. No fever. He had an ear infection 1 month ago. No current cough, runny nose, or nasal congestion. He is otherwise healthy and eating well. He was seen by his pediatrician this afternoon, but his ear was not infected. What is the cause of Eddie's ear pain?

Eddie has a serous otitis media with effusion, which is also known as an ear effusion or fluid in the ear. During an otoscope (ear) exam, you can see clear bubbles behind the tympanic membrane (TM/eardrum) in the middle ear space. There is no redness, bulging of the eardrum, or purulent (pus-containing) fluid. It can take weeks to months for the fluid to resolve. You may ask why Eddie has pain if there is no infection. Any fluid in the ear can be painful because it creates an uncomfortable pressure-like pain. Treatment is giving pain medication such as acetaminophen or ibuprofen.

Should Eddie go to the urgent care center tonight?

No. Eddie saw his pediatrician a few hours ago and there were no new changes.

Final Care Plan: Eddie used ibuprofen as needed and the pain resolved in 36 hours. Parents were advised to follow up with his pediatrician or go to urgent care if there is no improvement in 2-3 days or immediately if symptoms worsen.

Otitis Externa (Outer Ear Infection/Swimmer's Ear)

Nadia is a 10-year-old girl who started complaining of mild right ear pain yesterday. She noticed discharge on her pillow when she woke up earlier today. No fever, cough, runny nose, or nasal congestion. Nadia's family returned home today from a one-week vacation in Hawaii. Nadia last swam 2 days ago. What happened to Nadia?

Nadia has an acute otitis externa, which is also known as swimmer's ear. Otitis externa is different from otitis media (middle ear infection) because the ear canal becomes infected instead of the TM (eardrum). The TM usually looks normal. Otitis externa is also known as swimmer's ear because frequent swimming is one of its most common causes. Swimming can inadvertently flush earwax out of the ear. Ear wax helps prevent particles from getting inside of the ear.

During the otoscope exam, pulling the ear causes pain. Placing the otoscope tip into the inflamed canal can also cause extreme discomfort. The canal may be full of discharge, which can flow out of the ear. You may see this discharge on your child's pillowcase. Occasionally, there is so much discharge that the eardrum cannot be visualized.

How do we treat otitis externa? We use antibiotic otic (ear) drops such as Ciprodex (ciprofloxacin), Floxin (ofloxacin), and Cortisporin (neomycin, polymyxin B, and hydrocortisone). Acetaminophen and ibuprofen are used to treat the ear pain.

Should Nadia go?

Yes. Nadia needs to have her ears checked with an otoscope.

Final Care Plan: On exam, Nadia had pain when her ear was pulled to stretch the canal. Her canal was red, swollen, and had a whitish discharge. The TM was normal. Nadia was prescribed Floxin otic drops, and her ear pain resolved in 3 days.

Asthma

Olivia is an 8-year-old girl who has been coughing for the past 7 days. Last night, she started wheezing and complained that her chest felt tight. Although Olivia was wheezing, she did not have heavy breathing. Olivia also had a runny nose and nasal congestion when the cough started, but they both resolved 3 days ago. No fever, abdominal pain, vomiting or rash. She used her Albuterol inhaler once last night and once this morning. Both treatments provided relief that lasted at least 6 hours. Olivia has had similar episodes since she was 3 years old. What is causing these episodes?

Olivia is having an asthma exacerbation that was triggered from a viral URI. Asthma is a lower respiratory condition where small airways called bronchioles spasm or narrow and fill with mucus, which causes difficulty breathing. Each bronchiole ends with an air sac called an alveolus. Oxygen and carbon dioxide gas exchange takes place in the alveoli. When mucus plugs block bronchioles, the local alveoli beyond the blockages deflate and collapse. Blood oxygen levels fall because gas exchange cannot occur. This partial or complete lung segment collapse is called atelectasis.

Atelectasis can be seen on a chest x-ray and confirmed with a bronchoscopy. A bronchoscopy is a procedure used to visualize the inside of the lungs by inserting a tube with a camera on the end through the nose or mouth until it reaches the lungs. Lung imaging is not necessary to diagnose asthma but can be useful in detecting atelectasis.

Cough is the primary symptom of asthma. This cough may only occur at night, appear seasonally, or present in response to a specific trigger. A chronic cough that lasts for more than 3 weeks should raise suspicion for asthma. Examples of asthma triggers include allergens (e.g., dust, pollen, cigarette smoke, or cockroaches), illness (i.e., cold-induced asthma), or exercise.

Wheezing is the most recognized symptom that is associated with asthma. During an asthma exacerbation, air gets trapped inside of the tight airways. Wheezing is a noise that is appreciated when a breath is exhaled out of these tight bronchioles. Cough and wheezing often occur concurrently during an asthma exacerbation, but wheezing is not always necessary every time. Some may only wheeze occasionally, while others may not wheeze at all. The latter have cough-variant asthma. Your child may also start breathing faster.

As the breathing becomes more labored, you may notice retractions and nasal flaring. Retractions are when muscles in the neck, ribs, and abdomen assist breathing. When retractions are present, you can see these accessory muscles pull during each breath. Therefore, you should always look at your child's bare chest and abdomen when you notice any difficulty breathing. If the neck muscles are affected, the neck looks like it is tenting inward during the breath. When the rib muscles pull inward, the individual rib outlines become pronounced. If the abdominal muscles are affected, you will see the lower rib margin as the abdomen caves inward. Normally, the abdomen expands during inhalation as air enters the lungs. Abdominal retractions are noticed first because of the inward caving in the opposite direction. Nasal flaring is when the nostrils spread open while breathing.

Asthma is treated with medications categorized as rapid-acting/rescue medications vs. maintenance/controller medications. Ventolin/ProAir (albuterol) is an example of a rescue medication and has that designation because it has a rapid onset. Relief can be within minutes. Albuterol works by causing the tight bronchioles to dilate. It can be given as often as every 4 hours. If another dose is required sooner than 4 hours from the last dose, you should seek medical attention. Albuterol can be given continuously, if necessary, but this should be done with medical supervision.

Albuterol is prescribed in the nebulization or inhaler form. Oral albuterol is no longer recommended. When given via a nebulizer, the medicine is a liquid that comes in a vial, which is poured into a small reservoir called an acorn. The acorn has attachments for either a mask or a mouthpiece. Tubing connects the acorn to the nebulizer, which is a machine that causes the medication to be delivered in a mist-like state.

When given via an inhaler, the inhaler should be inserted into a cylindrical tube called an aerochamber or spacer. The other side of the inhaler should have a mask or mouthpiece depending on the age of the patient. An aerochamber serves as a reservoir where the medication remains, which allows the user to take several breaths to receive the entire dose. When using an Albuterol HFA inhaler WITHOUT an aerochamber, the user shakes the inhaler to mix the contents, presses down on the pump, takes a deep breath, and holds the breath for 10 seconds. This is not efficient for a few reasons. First, most people including adults do not coordinate their breathing as well as they think they do. Second, it is difficult to take a deep breath when there is chest tightness. If the user is unable to take a full breath, the inhaled medication may not even reach the lungs and only hit the back of the throat. Third, it is difficult to maintain that inhalation for the full 10 seconds if the user is coughing or short of breath.

When albuterol is given WITH an aerochamber, the user can take several breaths to ensure that the full dose is delivered. I recommend 5 breaths per puff where the inhaler is shaken prior to every puff. At 2 puffs per dose, that is a total of 10 breaths.

*Medication Administration Tip

You should always try to have an Albuterol inhaler at every living residence and at school so that the rescue medication can be given as soon as possible. You can request that your child's Albuterol inhaler prescription dispense two inhalers at a time.

As with all medications, albuterol has side effects. The main side effects are tachycardia (increased heart rate) and palpitations (the sensation that the heart is racing, pounding, or skipping beats). Tremor is another side effect. There is a medication called Xopenex (levalbuterol), which is a chemical variation of albuterol. Both have equal bronchodilation, but the variation in the chemical composition of Xopenex can decrease the adverse effects seen in albuterol. Xopenex may be used as a substitution for those who are unable to tolerate albuterol. Xopenex is available in the nebulization and inhaler form.

Maintenance medications on the other hand, do not work right away. They have to build up in the body before they take effect. That can take several days. Examples of maintenance medications are inhaled corticosteroids aka ICS (e.g., Pulmicort/budesonide, Flovent/fluticasone, Asmanex/mometasone, QVAR/beclomethasone) and a non-steroidal oral medication called Singulair/montelukast. Singulair can also be used to treat allergic rhinitis because it decreases inflammation throughout the entire body. Corticosteroids are anti-inflammatory medicines that decrease swelling and mucus production.

Inhaled steroids come in nebulizer and inhaler form similar to albuterol. One side effect of using an ICS inhaler is that the powder formulation can cause a fungal infection in the mouth and throat called thrush. Using an aerochamber can help decrease the risk of thrush because the medication is inhaled all the way into the lungs instead of settling in the throat. For older children and adults, certain inhalers come in a breath-activated form. These inhalers do not have a powder formulation. Breath-activated inhalers should be used without an aerochamber. You should confirm whether your breath-activated inhaler needs to be shaken before use.

When asthma exacerbations become more severe, an oral steroid may be prescribed. Examples of oral steroids are Orapred (prednisolone) and Decadron (dexamethasone). Prednisolone lasts in the body for 12-24 hours. Hence, it is prescribed as a once or twice per day dosing and is usually given for 3-5 days. Decadron, however, lasts in the body for 36-72 hours. Therefore, a single dose of Decadron is usually sufficient, but an additional dose may be given when necessary. If your child is having significant respiratory distress to the point that it is difficult to complete a sentence and there is a concern for swallowing, steroids may be administered intramuscularly (an injection into a muscle) or intravenously (into a vein).

Atrovent (ipratropium) is another medication that may be used during an asthma exacerbation. It is normally given in a healthcare setting, but there are special cases when a pulmonologist (lung doctor) may approve it for home use. Atrovent is another type of rapid-onset bronchodilator, but it acts on different receptors than albuterol or Xopenex. It can be given as a combination medicine with albuterol. This combination is called Combivent or Duoneb.

When a child presents to an urgent care center or emergency room with an asthma exacerbation, the asthma protocol is to give up to 3 back-to-back treatments of albuterol or Combivent/Duoneb with reassessment after every treatment by repeating the vital signs, lung exam, and heart exam. Reassessments are performed because the symptoms may resolve before all 3 treatments are given and we try not to administer unnecessary medicine. However, your child may receive all 3 treatments without reassessment if it was deemed that the exacerbation was severe. If the wheezing or cough has not improved, an oral steroid will likely be given. In order to be discharged home, the oxygen saturation should be at least 92% to 93% without requiring oxygen. The respiratory rate (i.e. breathing rate) should also be within a normal elevated range for age. Wheezing may not completely resolve, but there needs to be a significant improvement and close follow-up by your child's pediatrician or pulmonologist.

There is still some stigma associated with an asthma diagnosis. Hence, there is denial. People have come up with other terms such as reactive airway disease (RAD), allergic bronchitis, or recurrent pneumonia. Asthma is normally diagnosed around the age of 3 but can be diagnosed earlier if symptoms are consistent with asthma. RAD is often used when infants and toddlers present with symptoms consistent with asthma, but the diagnosis is unclear. When children continue to be diagnosed with RAD into their childhood years, the likely diagnosis is asthma.

Bronchitis is different than asthma because bronchitis is inflammation of the bronchi, which are the two larger airways that split off from the trachea (windpipe). Bronchitis is usually a diagnosis for adults. Once again, asthma affects the bronchioles, which are the smaller airways. Bacterial pneumonia does not occur repeatedly in a person who is not immunocompromised. Viral pneumonia can, however, trigger exacerbations, and in those cases, antibiotics are unnecessary.

In order to make a diagnosis of asthma in children, a careful review of current symptoms, past medical history, and family history needs to be performed in addition to at least one examination of your child. A history of symptoms consistent with asthma PLUS a finding of wheezing on exam strongly points to an asthma diagnosis.

In many cases, asthma can be diagnosed and treated by your pediatrician. However, if the diagnosis is unclear or the symptoms are poorly controlled, your child will be referred to a pulmonologist. Specialized lung tests called pulmonary function tests (PFTs) may be needed to diagnose asthma and rule out other possible causes. Spirometry is an example of a pulmonary function test. PFTs are performed by a pulmonologist. Another test is a peak expiratory flow rate. If your child was diagnosed with asthma, he or she may have a peak flow meter. This meter is used to track how well the asthma is being controlled. By having your child blow into the meter daily and more often when having an asthma exacerbation, you will be able to see when there is a change. PFTs and peak flows are less reliable in children under 6 years of age because they have difficulty following the instructions to properly perform the tests. In some cases, your child may be given a trial of albuterol to confirm the diagnosis. Albuterol is a medication that only works when there is a spasming of the bronchioles. Your child will not have any relief if the airways are fully open.

Once a diagnosis is confirmed, the severity of the illness is classified based on the symptom frequency. See Table 1.

Should Olivia go? No. The asthma exacerbation started yesterday is being managed well with Albuterol. She does not require any other medications at this time. Olivia should be seen immediately if she starts requiring Albuterol sooner than every 4 hours. She should follow up with her pediatrician if there is no improvement in 2-3 days.

Final Care Plan: Olivia continued to use her Albuterol inhaler via aerochamber every 4-6 hours and started to feel better by the third day.

Should We Go to Urgent Care?

		2 days per week MAX	More than 2 days per week but NOT daily	Daily	Throughout the day
IMPAIRMENT	Daytime symptom frequency	2 days per week MAX	More than 2 days per week but NOT daily	Daily	Throughout the day
	Nighttime awakenings	2 nights per month MAX	3-4 nights per month	More than 1 night per month	Every night
	SABA RESCUE med use (NOT counting pre-exercise)	2 days per week MAX	More than 2 days per week but NOT daily	Daily	Several times per day
	Activity limitation*	None	Minor	Some	Extreme
RISK	Attacks requiring oral steroids	0-1 time per year	At least 2 episodes in 12 months		
Severity classification	Severity classified based on the **WORST** columns above	INTERMITTENT	MILD PERSISTENT	MODERATE PERSISTENT	SEVERE PERSISTENT

Assess Severity of Symptoms over the past 4 weeks

SABA = short acting beta agonist (e.g. Albuterol, levalbuterol/Xopenex)

*Activity limitation is more often a symptom of poor control and NOT exercise-induced asthma

Eczema

Ian is a 13-year-old boy with a history of dry skin who has been complaining of itchiness for 1 week. He has dry, red, scaly patches on his hands, elbows, knees, and abdomen. He has been scratching constantly. No fever, headache, ear pain, sore throat, cough, runny nose, congestion, vomiting, or diarrhea. No new foods, medications, clothing, soap, laundry detergent, or lotions. Ian denies going into any wooded areas or playing in bushes. When asked, Ian reports that he does not use skin moisturizers. Ian's mother reports that he gets recurrent episodes of itchiness. What is Ian's diagnosis?

Ian has eczema aka atopic dermatitis. Eczema is a chronic skin condition that causes it to become dry, itchy, red, and inflamed. The rash can present in infancy or early childhood. In older children, the rash appears as dry, scaly patches in skin creases such as in front of the elbows or behind the knees. It can also be seen on the face, behind the neck, on the abdomen, and on the hands. The patches do not have a particular shape unless the eczema is a form called nummular eczema. That form of eczema looks like coin-shaped patches and can be mistaken for ringworm. The rash can appear to wax and wane over time. When the rash worsens, it is referred to as an eczema exacerbation or flare. The rash can be triggered by a dry environment, cold weather, wind, rapid temperature changes, sweating, dust, sand, and even cigarette smoke. Certain soaps, detergents, lotions, perfumes, synthetic fibers, and wool can also irritate the skin.

The most important treatment for eczema is frequent moisturization to prevent the skin from drying out. Bathing should be limited to 10 minutes (no more than 15 minutes) and the water should be lukewarm instead of hot because hot water and prolonged bathing can dry out the skin. Gentle, hypoallergenic cleaners without fragrances such as Cetaphil should be used, and scrubbing the skin should be avoided. You should also stay away from antibacterial cleansers. After bathing, pat the skin dry instead of rubbing the skin. This will leave the skin slightly damp.

Next, the skin should be moisturized immediately with a thick lotion, cream, or ointment to prevent the skin from drying out as the water evaporates. Eucerin, Aveeno, Aquaphor, Cetaphil, Nivea, and CeraVe are good options for daily lotions or creams and are available over-the-counter at your local drugstore or grocery store. They have thicker ointment options that come in round tub containers. Petroleum jelly or Vaseline can also be used as an ointment. Use the thickness that suits your child best. The skin should be moisturized at least twice per day and more often, if necessary, especially after your child was sweating or participated in a water activity.

When treating an eczema exacerbation, you may be advised to apply topical steroid cream or ointment such as hydrocortisone 1-2 times per day. Daily use is not suggested unless your child was referred to a dermatologist who gave that recommendation because prolonged daily steroid use can thin the skin. In severe cases, a short course of oral steroids may be prescribed. If these initial treatments do not help, your child may be referred to a dermatologist.

Should Ian go?

Yes. He should have a skin examination to determine whether prescription medications are necessary. Due to the constant skin dryness and scratching, the skin can become infected. During the skin exam, Ian should also be checked for any signs of local infection.

Final Care Plan: Ian had several red, inflamed, dry, scaly skin patches. The skin was not infected. Ian was prescribed a 7-day course of prescription-strength steroid cream. He was also advised to start moisturizing his skin at least twice per day.

Allergic Rhinitis (Seasonal Allergies/Hay Fever)

Scott is a 10-year-old boy who has an 8-day history of sneezing, runny nose, nasal congestion, nasal itchiness, and eye itchiness. His eyes are watery and red, but there is no discharge. He is also complaining of intermittent headaches, pressure in his cheeks, and ear stuffiness. He has been clearing his throat because of reported throat itchiness. No wheezing, chest tightness, abdominal pain, vomiting, diarrhea, or rash. He is eating well. Scott has these symptoms every springtime and takes a medication that provides relief, but parents are unsure of the medication name. Why is Scott having these symptoms?

Scott has allergic rhinitis. The sinuses are air-filled cavities inside the face that also have a mucosal lining. This mucosal lining extends into the nose and goes down to the lungs, coating the entire respiratory tract. The lining normally produces mucus, which traps dust, smoke, bacteria, and other small particles. It also prevents the linings from drying out. This mucus is unknowingly swallowed throughout the day. There is also a mucosal lining that coats the entire digestive system but lacks cilia. Cilia are hair-like projections that either move mucus from the nasal passages or the lungs toward the throat where it can be swallowed or spit out.

Rhinitis is inflammation of the mucus membrane lining inside the nasal passages. When the passages become inflamed, excess mucus is produced and the linings become swollen. This swelling causes nasal congestion. As the swelling worsens, the sinuses are no longer able to drain their mucus into the nose. This can create pressure or fullness in the sinuses. The excess mucus can flow forward out of the nose, causing a runny nose. If it travels to the back of the nose and down the throat, older children and adults can spit this excess mucus out. Otherwise, the excess mucus is swallowed.

When the cause is allergic, rhinitis is classified as allergic rhinitis and is caused by substances called allergens. Examples of these inhaled substances are dust, pollen, ragweed, mold, or pet dander. The body recognizes these allergens as being foreign and stimulates the immune system to react. This starts a reaction where mast cells release histamine. Eye involvement can occur with allergic rhinitis and is specifically called allergic conjunctivitis. With allergic conjunctivitis, the conjunctivae (linings that coat the eyeball) are red and itchy. There may be excessive tearing or watery discharge but pooling purulent (greenish or yellowish pus-like discharge) discharge is not seen. Purulent discharge is with bacterial conjunctivitis, which we discussed in a previous section.

Sneezing is an involuntary action that occurs to remove irritants from your nose and throat. The excess mucus can cause throat itchiness or soreness, but most do not complain of pain with swallowing. On exam, "allergic shiners" may be appreciated, and you may notice your child doing the "allergic salute." Allergic shiners are bluish-gray to purple discolorations under the eyes. The eyelids may be swollen, but there is no associated tenderness to touch. The allergic salute is the movement seen when one repeatedly rubs the nose and pushes the tip of the nose up with the hand in response to nasal itching. This upwards salute causes a horizontal crease over the nose.

Many people do not think that it is necessary to treat allergy symptoms. This is a false notion. When allergic rhinitis goes untreated, not only does your child have to deal with the nasal, eye, and throat symptoms, but chronic nasal congestion can cause headaches and decreased sleep. Decreased sleep leads to daytime sleepiness and poor concentration. In children, you may also see behavioral changes and irritability.

Allergic rhinitis is treated with different medications. The first medication is an antihistamine, which blocks the histamine reaction from occurring. Oral Antihistamines come in liquid and pill form. Examples of antihistamines are Benadryl/diphenhydramine, Claritin (loratadine), Zyrtec (cetirizine), and Allegra (fexofenadine). Benadryl (diphenhydramine) is one of the earlier antihistamines created. It works well and can be given to all ages including babies, but the main side effect is drowsiness. Claritin, Zyrtec, and Allegra are newer medicines that are in a different class. They can also cause drowsiness but to a much lesser extent.

For children ages 12 and older, there is a class of allergy medicines that is a combination of an antihistamine and a decongestant. It only comes in pill form. Examples of this class of medication are Claritin-D (loratadine-D), Zyrtec-D (cetirizine-D), and Allegra-D (fexofenadine-D). They are available without a prescription but are behind the pharmacist's counter. A government-issued photo ID must be provided to purchase this medication.

In addition to oral antihistamines, there are allergy nasal sprays and eye drops. Both the nasal and eye medicines can be divided into antihistamine and steroid medicines. In the pediatric world, allergy eye drops are usually limited to antihistamines. Antihistamine eye drops prevent Examples of antihistamine allergy eye drops are Zaditor (ketotifen), azelastine, epinastine (Elestat), and Patanol/Pataday (olopatadine hydrochloride).

Examples of antihistamine nasal sprays include Astelin/Astepro (azelastine) and Patanase (olopatadine). Examples of steroid nasal sprays are Flonase (fluticasone), Nasacort (triamcinolone), Nasonex (mometasone), Rhinocort (budesonide), and Qnasl (beconase).

*Medication Administration Tip

When using nasal sprays, assist or direct your child in blowing his or her nose and shaking the bottle before spraying. Blowing the nose helps clear any mucus. You need to be mindful of two things: first, the pump is primed, and second, you are holding the pump in the correct position. You need to prime the pump for its initial use and re-prime it if you have not used it in 7 days. When priming the pump for its first use, remove the cap, point it away from any faces, and push down on the pump 8-10 times until a fine mist is seen. To re-prime the pump, you may only need to press down on the pump 2 or 3 times until a fine mist is seen. Once the pump is primed, insert it into one nostril pointing it slightly outward aiming toward the outer corner of the eye, cover the opposite nostril with a finger, and have your child inhale as the pump is being pressed down to release the medicine. Pointing the pump outward increases medication delivery because it is pointed toward the sinuses in your cheek. Pointing the pump toward the middle of the face will spray the septum, which is made of cartilage and is not involved when there is nasal congestion. Pointing the pump straight back will increase drippage of the spray down the throat.

Other useful home remedies include using a nasal saline spray, a cool-mist humidifier, steamy showers, and saltwater gargles.

NOTE: You need to be careful with over-the-counter nasal decongestant sprays like Afrin/oxymetazoline because if you use them for longer than 3 days in a row, they can cause a rebound effect, which is when the nasal passages become congested once again.

Should Scott go?

No. Scott has a history of allergic rhinitis, which is relieved by allergy medications. Bacterial sinusitis is not a concern at this time, so antibiotics do not need to be started.

Final Care Plan: Scott's mother made an appointment the following day with his pediatrician for an allergy follow-up visit where he can restart his allergy medications. While home that evening, Scott was given a nasal saline spray and used the cool-mist humidifier. The headache was relieved with ibuprofen. The throat itchiness was relieved by saltwater gargles and lots of fluids.

Anaphylaxis

Lauren is a 7-year-old girl who accompanied her family to a Sunday brunch. She ordered fried shrimp, French fries, and an orange soda. This was her first time eating shrimp. About 30 minutes later, Lauren's face, lips, tongue, and eyelids became swollen. Lauren became frightened because her throat felt tight and itchy. Her body broke out into hives. What is happening to Lauren?

Lauren is having an anaphylactic reaction. Anaphylaxis is defined as a rapid onset (minutes to several hours) severe allergic reaction that affects 2 or more organ systems. Organ systems can be broken down into:

1. Skin/mucosal tissue

    a. Hives (welt-like rash) all over the body

    b. Itchy, flushed skin

    c. eyelid, lip, or tongue swelling

    d. pale or bluish color

2. Respiratory

    a. shortness of breath or labored breathing

    b. throat tightness with difficulty swallowing or speaking

    c. wheezing

    d. stridor

    e. low levels of oxygen in the blood

3. Gastrointestinal (GI or digestive) – these symptoms are persistent

   a. crampy abdominal pain

   b. vomiting with or without nausea

   c. diarrhea

4. Cardiovascular (circulatory)

   a. Reduced blood pressure

   b. Syncope (fainting)

   c. Incontinence (lack of voluntary control over urination or defecation)

In addition to the criteria stated above, other symptoms occur with anaphylaxis. These include rapid onset of runny nose, nasal congestion, throbbing headache, tunnel vision, dizziness, lightheadedness, or confusion. Your child may become anxious or irritable. Younger children may have a sudden behavioral change. Older children and adults sometimes verbalize this "sense of impending doom" as feeling like they are going to die.

The most important thing to remember with anaphylaxis is that giving epinephrine as soon as possible prevents the progression to life-threatening symptoms, including shock. If your child was prescribed an EpiPen and there is a concern for anaphylaxis, it is advised that you administer the EpiPen immediately, note the time that it was given, and then take your child for medical evaluation and observation. Your child needs to be observed for 4-6 hours after contact with the offending agent to ensure that the symptoms do not return.

*Medication Administration Tip

Ask your pediatrician or allergist to prescribe two EpiPens at a time so that you can keep one at your child's school.

Should Lauren go? Yes. Even if the EpiPen is administered outside of a medical facility, your child should always be evaluated and observed afterward.

Final Care Plan: Lauren was given epinephrine and Benadryl in the office. Since it was still early in the day, Lauren was able to complete her 6-hour observation at the urgent care center. If the office were closing, Lauren would have been referred to the local emergency room to complete her observation period there. After completing the observation period, Lauren was discharged home. The family had Claritin at home and used it as needed for itching since it is a once-per-day dosing and it causes less drowsiness than Benadryl. Zyrtec and Allegra are other options instead of Claritin. Lauren's mother was advised to wait at least 4 weeks before getting allergy testing because it takes a few weeks for new histamine creation to replace what was released during the histamine release. If you do allergy testing too early, your child may falsely test negative.

Croup

Tommy is a 4-year-old boy who woke up overnight with a barky cough. He started having temps to 101.3°F, runny nose, and cough earlier in the day, but his cough was not barky at that time. Tommy started crying when he woke up coughing. His voice was hoarse, and he had noisy breathing with inhalation. After calming down, the noisy breathing resolved. He is not breathing fast or hard. No headache, ear pain, sore throat, abdominal pain, vomiting, diarrhea, or rash. Tommy only ate a small amount of his dinner but has been drinking well throughout the day. What causes a barky cough?

Tommy has viral croup. The medical term for croup is laryngotracheitis because the larynx (voice box) and trachea (windpipe) are affected. Croup is seen mostly in the winter months and affects children between 3 months and 5 years of age. Some children continue to have episodes of croup through their later childhood, but most children grow out of the symptoms because their airways grow along with the rest of their bodies, and the larger lumen (i.e., a channel within a tube) can have narrowing without affecting the cough or breathing. In most cases, croup lasts for about 3 days before resolving on its own. Viral croup is caused by different viruses including parainfluenzae (different from the flu), respiratory syncytial virus (RSV), measles adenovirus, and influenza (the flu virus). It is diagnosed clinically, which means that the diagnosis is made from the history presented by the parent and the physical exam findings.

The most associated symptom is a barking cough. The cough becomes barky when the air passes through the inflamed and narrowed opening. As the airway tightens, your child may develop stridor. Stridor is a noise appreciated when your child inhales. When there is mild airway narrowing, stridor may only be appreciated when your child is crying or active, but it resolves when your child is comfortably at rest. That is a reassuring sign that the airway tightness is not severe. If, however, stridor is present when your child is comfortably at rest, this is a medical emergency. Your child should be evaluated immediately. Fever and runny nose may also be seen.

Croup is treated with steroids to decrease inflammation. Similar to asthma treatment, the steroids are usually administered by mouth, but if your child is having significant respiratory distress, the medication may be given as an injection into a muscle. The drug of choice is a single dose of Decadron (dexamethasone). If Decadron is not available, your child will receive a dose of Orapred (prednisolone) in the office or ER with a prescription for the following 2 days to complete a 3-day course.

If your child is having stridor while comfortably at rest, racemic epinephrine is given via the nebulizer. If your child is given a Racemic Epi nebulization treatment, expect there to be an observation period of 2-4 hours to ensure that the stridor does not recur. Racemic EPI nebs are not prescribed for home use.

The goal of the treatments is to keep the child as comfortable as possible. Avoiding agitation can decrease crying. Humidified air is the primary treatment. It is wise to own a humidifier because it is easier to breathe humidified air versus dry air. Cool mist humidifiers are preferred, but warm humidity is better than none. If you do not have access to a humidifier, other options are useful. Sitting in a steamy bathroom for 20 minutes or walking outside in the cooler air can provide temporary relief. Another method is sticking your child's head in front of an open freezer for a few minutes. Be sure your child is wearing appropriate layers for the colder options.

Should Tommy go?

Yes. He needs to be evaluated today. If his pediatrician is unable to schedule a sick visit today, an urgent care center is a good option. Tommy needs to have his vital signs assessed to measure his temperature and respiratory rate. If possible, his oxygen saturation can also be measured. Tommy should also have a heart and lung exam at the very minimum.

Final Care Plan: At the start of the exam, Tommy was scared and began to cry. While crying, stridor was appreciated while he was breathing. The stridor resolved once he calmed down. Tommy had a barky cough. His temp was 101 °F, respiratory rate was slightly elevated at 28 breaths per minute, and O_2 sat was 97%. Lungs were clear and he did not have retractions. Tommy was given one oral dose of Decadron and sent home with instructions to use his cool mist humidifier and give acetaminophen as needed for fever or discomfort. His symptoms resolved in 2 days.

Typical (Classic) Pneumonia

Devin is a 6-year-old boy who presents with a 5-day history of fevers to 103 °F, chills, and a 2-day history of a loose cough. He appears tired and has been breathing slightly faster than usual. No wheezing. No headache, ear pain, sore throat, abdominal pain, vomiting, diarrhea, or rash. Devin has a poor appetite but will have small amounts of soup and juice when encouraged. No previous history of wheezing. Why isn't Devin improving?

Devin has typical community-acquired pneumonia. Pneumonia is inflammation of the lung tissue caused by bacterial, viral, or fungal infections. This inflammation causes alveoli (air sacs located at the end of bronchioles where oxygen and carbon dioxide gas exchange is made while breathing) to fill up with fluid or pus. Community-acquired means that the infection was contracted in the community vs nosocomial (hospital-acquired) pneumonia. Pneumonia is described as typical when it is caused by certain bacteria that commonly cause this illness. These bacteria cause infections in a lobar distribution, which means that there is a fluid infiltrate in at least one lung lobe. This localized consolidation may be visualized on a chest x-ray, but x-rays are not always necessary.

Streptococcus pneumoniae is the most common cause of bacterial pneumonia in children. *Haemophilus influenzae* type b (Hib) is the second most common cause of pneumonia. Vaccination helps prevent these infections.

The pneumococcal (Prevnar) and Hib vaccines are given, respectively.

Signs and symptoms of pneumonia include fever, chills, cough, increased respiratory rate, shallow breathing, shortness of breath, sharp or stabbing chest pain with breathing (seen in older children and adults), fatigue, sweating, and loss of appetite. Fever and difficulty breathing may present prior to the cough because it takes time for the cough receptors in the alveoli to be activated by the infection. Occasionally, abdominal pain may be a symptom due to referred pain from the lower lobes of the lungs.

Many pneumonia diagnoses are made based on the clinical exam. During a lung exam, breath sounds are diminished where the fluid is present. In addition to the air flow being diminished, your pediatrician may report hearing fluid in the lungs while listening with a stethoscope. This sound is called crackles or rales because the air moving through the fluid produces intermittent, crackling noises. If the lung exam is unclear and no source of infection (e.g. ear, throat, sinuses, lungs, urine, etc.) is identified, a chest x-ray may be warranted.

Your child's respiratory rate and heart rate may be elevated, but it should be within the accepted range for your child's age. The oxygen saturation should be at least 92% to 93% without the need for supplemental oxygen. Your child's breathing should not be labored. Crackles and/ or decreased breath sounds are sufficient to make a clinical diagnosis of pneumonia. If those breath sounds are appreciated, a chest x-ray is unnecessary. After a full physical exam is performed, it can be determined whether your child can go home on antibiotics and close follow-up or if referral to a local emergency room is necessary

Antibiotic treatment for typical pneumonia is similar to the treatment for otitis media because the bacterial causes are the same. The treatment of choice is a 7-day course of high-dose amoxicillin. If your child has a mild amoxicillin allergy (not anaphylaxis), you can treat with Omnicef/cefdinir. If your child has a severe amoxicillin allergy, other antibiotic options include clindamycin, clarithromycin/Biaxin, and levofloxacin/Levaquin. Improvement should be seen in 2-3 days, but the cough and fatigue may persist for weeks to months after the initial infection. You may treat the fever with acetaminophen or ibuprofen.

Should Devin go?

Yes. Devin needs an in-person evaluation to check his vital signs, lungs, and heart.

Final Care Plan: Devin's respiratory rate was 32 breaths per minute and his oxygen saturation was 93% on room air. He had mild retractions. Crackles and decreased breath sounds were appreciated in the right lower lobe during the lung exam. Devin was discharged home and prescribed a 7-day course of high-dose amoxicillin. His parents monitored his symptoms closely and continued to encourage fluids. Acetaminophen was given for fever and discomfort. Ibuprofen was given sparingly when Devin's parents convinced to eat a small amount of food. Devin had a follow-up appointment with his pediatrician the following afternoon. Devin's respiratory rate decreased to 28 breaths per minute, his retractions resolved, and his oxygen saturation was 95% on room air. His fever resolved in 48 hours. Devin continued to have fatigue for the next week but otherwise improved.

Atypical (Walking) Pneumonia

Kelly is an 11-year-old girl who had a dry cough, runny nose, headache, sore throat, and fevers to 100.8°F for 4 days. She was seen by her pediatrician on Day 4 of illness where Strep and flu testing was negative. The heart and lung exams were negative at that time. All symptoms resolved within the next 3 days, but the cough began to worsen. Kelly has now been coughing for a total of days. Her appetite is slightly decreased, but she is still eating and drinking fluids. Although she had not been feeling well, Kelly was able to play when she was afebrile. What is the diagnosis?

Kelly has atypical pneumonia aka walking pneumonia. As discussed in the previous chapter, pneumonia is inflammation of the lung tissue caused by bacterial, viral, or fungal infections. This inflammation causes alveoli (air sacs located at the end of bronchioles where oxygen and carbon dioxide gas exchange is made while breathing) to fill up with fluid or pus.

Atypical pneumonia is another type of community-acquired pneumonia (i.e., contracted in the community vs. in a hospital setting). It is commonly referred to as walking pneumonia because you are not as ill-appearing as when you have classic or typical pneumonia. Your child likely will not require bed rest and could be "walking around" with everyone unaware of the lung infection.

Both types of pneumonia will present with fever, cough, difficulty breathing, abnormal breath sounds, and fatigue, but the symptoms are less severe in atypical pneumonia. Fevers are low grade and there may be mild difficulty breathing. Chills, sweats, and an ill appearance are primarily seen in typical pneumonia.

The main distinguishing symptom in atypical pneumonia is that the cough is usually nonproductive (dry) and it progressively worsens. This cough may persist for weeks to months. Given that atypical pneumonia can produce a more diffuse, patchy infiltration, crackles and decreased breath sounds may be heard in more than one region of one or both lungs. If a chest x-ray is obtained, this patchy distribution may be seen. Of note, atypical pneumonia may also cause a focal consolidation similar to what is seen in typical lobar pneumonia so x-ray results are not definitive. The culmination of findings from your child's history, physical exam, and optional chest x-ray is used to formulate a final diagnosis. Bloodwork may also be obtained to test for bacterial antibodies, but this is only performed when warranted.

Mycoplasma pneumoniae is the most common bacteria that causes atypical pneumonia. In addition to the symptoms stated above, it may also present with a runny nose, headache, rash, and wheezing. Not only can a mycoplasma infection worsen asthma symptoms, but it can also cause wheezing in children who do not have a history of asthma.

The antibiotic of choice for mycoplasmal pneumonia is Zithromax (azithromycin). This is different than amoxicillin or cephalosporin choices used to treat typical bacteria. The azithromycin course is 5 days with a big dose on Day 1 and 4 smaller doses for days 2-5. If your child has an azithromycin allergy, other antibiotic options are Biaxin (clarithromycin), doxycycline, erythromycin, and tetracycline. Tetracycline is only recommended as an option for children who are at least 8 years of age. Albuterol may be recommended if your child is wheezing. Acetaminophen and ibuprofen should still be used to treat fever and pain. Improvement should be seen in 2-3 days.

Should Kelly go?

Yes. Given the duration of symptoms and the worsening cough, Kelly should have another in-person evaluation to see if there are any other changes on exam such as increasing respiratory or heart rate, decreasing oxygen saturation, and abnormal heart or lung sounds.

Final Care Plan: Kelly's respiratory rate was slightly elevated at 26 breaths per minute and her oxygen saturation was 96% on room air. Crackles were appreciated in both sides of the chest during the lung exam. No wheezing or rash was appreciated. She was discharged home and prescribed azithromycin. Cough started to improve within 48 hours, but it lingered for another week.

COVID-19

Will is a 12-year-old boy with fever (T_{max} 100.8°), cough, headache, sore throat, vomiting, diarrhea, and body aches for the past 3 days. He vomited once per day and had 2 episodes of watery stool. He does not have any difficulty breathing. Today, he reported that he was no longer able to smell or taste his food. He has been eating soup and crackers. He is tolerating fluids. No known sick contacts, but Will did return to in-school learning 1 month ago. What does Will have? What distinguishes this illness from the flu?

Will has COVID-19. Coronaviruses were identified in the 1960s. They cause viral URI (common cold) symptoms like cough, runny nose, and nasal congestion. In 2019, a novel coronavirus was identified, which caused severe pneumonia. This disease process was named COVID-19 or coronavirus 2019. The virus that causes COVID-19 is named SARS-CoV-2, which stands for severe acute respiratory syndrome coronavirus 2. It is transmitted from person to person through respiratory droplets. In March 2020, the World Health Organization declared COVID-19 a global pandemic. COVID-19 disproportionately affects children and adults from underrepresented racial and ethnic groups. This is likely due to living within close proximity to others in apartment buildings, living in multigenerational homes, poverty, family members who are essential workers, and limited access to healthcare.

Symptoms of COVID-19 appear 2-14 days after exposure from an infected person. Many of the symptoms seen in COVID-19 overlap with influenza symptoms. These include fever, cough, runny nose, shortness of breath, headache, sore throat, body aches, nausea, vomiting, diarrhea, and body aches. The main distinguishing symptom is that COVID-19 can cause anosmia, which is the medical term for loss of taste or smell. Anosmia is not necessary for a COVID-19 diagnosis, but if it is present, it increases the likelihood.

Active COVID-19 infection is confirmed using two different tests. Both are nasal swabs. One test is the rapid test. This test is similar to the Rapid Strep test that is looking for the antigen. Antigens are substances on a cell that cause the body to elicit an immune response to produce antibodies. The polymerase chain reaction (PCR) test is the most accurate. This test amplifies or makes copies of the virus if it is present. Therefore, a very small specimen can test positive. Antibody testing, on the other hand, tests for past infection. The body takes about 2 weeks to make antibodies against an antigen. Hence, positive antibodies will show a past infection.

Most treatment for COVID-19 is lots of rest and supportive care. Hospitalization is usually reserved for patients who require oxygen, have signs of altered mental status (e.g., confusion, agitation, decreased alertness, change in behavior, etc.), or signs of shock.

If your child tests positive and DOES have symptoms, he or she must be isolated from other family members as best as possible until:

1. At least 10 days since symptoms first appeared AND

2. At least 24 hours with no fever without fever-reducing medication (e.g., acetaminophen)

3. Other symptoms of COVID-19 are improving

*Loss of taste or smell is not a factor when it comes to ending isolation since it may persist for weeks or months after recovery

If your child tests positive and does NOT have symptoms, isolation must continue until after 10 days have passed since the last positive test.

If your child tests negative, but had close contact (e.g., within 6 feet for over 15 minutes) with a person who tested positive for COVID-19, your child should quarantine for:

1. 10-14 days without testing

OR

2. 7 days after receiving a negative test (test must occur on Day 5 or later)

Check with your local health department for criteria regarding ending quarantine early.

Currently, the Pfizer vaccine is available for children ages 12 and older. Vaccination is given in 2 doses that are administered 3 weeks apart. Your child will be considered fully vaccinated 2 weeks after the second vaccine.

Should Will go?

Yes. Will should have his vitals checked along with getting his heart, lungs, and abdomen checked.

Final Care Plan: Will had a temp of 100.7°, respiratory rate of breaths per minute, heart rate of 120 beats per minute, blood pressure of 110/70 mm Hg, and an O_2 sat of 98% on room air. He was stable to be discharged home and was placed on isolation. Parents monitored Will very closely for any signs of difficulty breathing or any other concerning symptoms. All of Will's symptoms resolved in 13 days except for the anosmia. His taste and smell did not return for 2 months. Will received the Pfizer vaccine 1 month later.

Acute Gastroenteritis (AGE, Stomach Flu)

Beth is an 11-year-old girl who had three episodes of vomiting and four episodes of non-bloody diarrhea since last night. Beth last vomited 1 hour ago. She is complaining of nausea and mild abdominal pain. No fever, headache, sore throat, or rash. Beth urinated twice today. What is the cause of her symptoms?

Beth has acute gastroenteritis (AGE), which is inflammation of the lining of the digestive tract. Although gastroenteritis is also known as "the stomach flu," it is not caused by influenza. Instead, it is caused by other viruses such as rotavirus, norovirus, and adenovirus. Common symptoms are diarrhea with or without vomiting, nausea, abdominal pain, and fever. Vomiting usually lasts 1-3 days. Diarrhea usually lasts 5-7 days but persists in some for up to 2 weeks.

The main treatment is rehydration. Rehydration is attempted by mouth first. After avoiding food and water for at least 30 minutes, children are started on a PO challenge. A PO challenge is performed to ensure fluids can be tolerated.

Clear fluids are preferred. Oral rehydration solutions like Pedialyte are the best option and can be given to all ages including babies because they are composed of water, electrolytes, and a small amount of sugar. When you have vomiting or diarrhea, you not only lose water, but you also lose electrolytes. However, Pedialyte is often not tolerated well by older children and adults because it is so salty.

Pedialyte ice pops are sometimes tolerated better than the liquid.

Gatorade and Powerade were created with a higher amount of sugar so that people will drink them. They are safe to drink once your child has been weaned off breast-milk or formula and is consuming a regular diet. Your child is at the age where water and flat ginger ale are also acceptable options because you do not have to be as care-ful with maintaining the electrolyte balance after infancy. If your child had excessive vomiting, foods should not be restarted until 6 hours after the last vomiting episode to give the digestive system time to rest.

Be careful to give clear fluids in small amounts starting at 5-10 milliliters (1-2 teaspoons) every 10 minutes. You can increase the amount by 5-10 milliliters (ml) every 15-30 minutes. For example, give 5ml (1 teaspoon) every 5 minutes for 15-30 minutes, then 10 ml every 5 minutes for 15-30 minutes. Continue to slowly increase the volume as tolerated.

Once nausea and vomiting are better for about 6-12 hours, try bland food such as saltine crackers, toast, dry cereal, rice, applesauce, or bananas. Chicken can be given, but it should be baked, and the skin should be removed. Avoid greasy, creamy, and spicy foods. Do not force foods. It is okay if your child does not eat solids for a few days as long as he or she can drink fluids.

If your child continues to vomit, he or she needs to have a medical evaluation to determine hydration status.

Anti-nausea medications like ondansetron/Zofran and metoclopramide/Reglan can be given during the evaluation if available. Ondansetron is more commonly given. Most pediatricians do not have anti-nausea medications or IV fluids in their offices. Therefore, evaluation at an urgent care center or a local emergency room is the preferred next step after a failed PO challenge at home.

After ondansetron is given, parents are advised to wait another 30 minutes before restarting the PO challenge. Your child is allowed to vomit one more time after receiving ondansetron. If your child continues to vomit thereafter, the PO challenge failed. Your child will need IV hydration and possible IV anti-nausea medication. Many urgent care centers are equipped to give IV fluids over a short period of time. If your child requires more than that one measured bolus of fluids, he or she will be transferred to an ER for further evaluation and care. Once the nausea resolves, a new PO challenge will be attempted.

Acetaminophen may be given as needed for fever or pain. Ibuprofen should be avoided because it can irritate the stomach. Antidiarrheal medications like Lomotil, Imodium/Kaopectate, and Pepto-Bismol are not recommended to treat infectious causes of diarrhea in children.

During a medical evaluation, your child may have blood, urine, or stool taken for testing or imaging (e.g., x-ray, ultrasound, CT scan) may be performed, but in most cases of viral acute gastroenteritis with mild dehydration, testing is unnecessary.

Viral AGEs can make your child uncomfortable, but they are still usually well appearing. Some symptoms require immediate evaluation. These symptoms include having a toxic/ill appearance (i.e., lethargy, paleness, bluish skin, or abnormal breathing), signs of dehydration (e.g., dry mouth, no tears when crying, no urine for over 8 hours), persistent vomiting, blood in the vomit, bile (bright green color) in the vomit, severe abdominal pain, blood in the stool, more than 8-10 stools per day) or fever lasting longer than 48 hours.

Should Beth go?

Yes. Beth should have her vital signs, throat, and abdomen checked. An increased heart rate and/or decreased blood pressure could be a sign of dehydration. Doing an abdominal exam can help rule out if there are any surgical concerns.

Final Care Plan: Heart rate was mildly elevated. Blood pressure was normal. No fever. Abdominal exam was normal. Beth was given ondansetron and advised to avoid eating or drinking anything for 30 minutes. Beth tolerated 4 ounces of Gatorade during her PO challenge and was discharged home.

Sickle Cell Disease (Sickle Cell Anemia)

Maria is a 12-year-old girl who had a sudden onset of severe pain in her shoulders, arms, back, hips, and legs starting this morning. The pain is debilitating, and she has been in bed crying throughout the day. No fever, cough, chest pain, shortness of breath, abdominal pain, vomiting, diarrhea, or rash. She has used ibuprofen and without relief. Maria takes hydroxyurea. No other meds. She has frequent pain episodes, most of which are managed at home. What is the cause of Maria's pain?

Maria has sickle cell disease (SCD). Sickle cell disease is a blood disorder where there is a gene mutation on a hemoglobin chain. This mutation causes the red blood cell (RBC) to change from its round doughnut-like shape to a sickle shape when oxygen levels are low. Sickle cell disease is also known as sickle cell anemia because it causes chronic anemia. Sickle cells are less flexible than normal RBCs. When blood flows, the cells flow freely as they travel in the bloodstream, bouncing off the vessel walls. When sickle cells hit these walls, their rigidity causes them to undergo hemolysis (i.e., rupture or destruction of RBCs). This hemolytic anemia causes hemoglobin levels to be approximately 7g/dl at baseline. Hemolytic anemia can also cause jaundice (i.e., yellowing of the skin and the whites of the eyes as a result of excessive RBC breakdown). Jaundice can become more pronounced as the anemia worsens.

In addition to hemolytic anemia, sickle cells are stickier than normal RBCs. They are unable to squeeze through smaller vessels and get trapped. The sickle cells begin to stack on each other and create a blockage. Blood cannot flow beyond the blockages. Oxygen travels on RBCs so it also gets trapped. There is subsequent tissue death beyond the clogged areas due to a lack of oxygen. This process is extremely painful and referred to as a vaso-occlusive pain episode.

Vaso-occlusive pain episodes can begin as early as 6 months of age and recur throughout life. One of the earliest symptoms seen is called dactylitis. Dactylitis is painful swelling of the hands and feet. Parents note that their child's fingers and toes look like red sausages. Dactylitis is seen between 6 months and 6 years of age. As the child gets older, pain sites can include the arms, legs, chest, back, and abdomen.

Sickle cell disease can affect any area of the body including the eyes (damage to the retina), gallbladder (gallstones), kidney (scarring that can lead to kidney failure), and skin (ulcers). In addition to the increase of overall infection, the risk of bone infection (osteomyelitis) is increased in sickle cell disease.

One of the most concerning complications is called Acute Chest Syndrome (ACS). ACS is diagnosed when a patient with sickle cell disease meets certain criteria:

1. a NEW lung infiltrate (collection of fluid or pus) seen on chest x-ray involving at least one complete

lung segment that is not consistent with the appearance of atelectasis (partial or complete lung collapse)

AND one or more of the following signs or symptoms:

2. chest pain

3. a temperature greater than $38.5°C = 101.3°F$

4. increased respiratory rate, wheezing, cough, or signs of increased work of breathing (e.g. retractions)

5. Hypoxemia (low blood oxygen levels) relative to oxygen levels at baseline when patient is healthy

Another complication is priapism, which is persistent, painful erections caused by sickle cells getting lodged in the blood vessels of the penis. Erections can present in either the "stuttering" fashion where the episodes are brief and may occur daily or in the "prolonged" fashion where erections last for over 4 hours. Prolonged episodes may cause permanent damage to the penis and possible impotence due to the decreased blood flow to the area for such long periods of time.

Splenic and hepatic sequestration may also occur. This is when the sickle cells become trapped in the spleen and liver, respectively. The liver and spleen filter the body's blood. Therefore, large amounts of blood travel through them daily. When sickle cells stack in the spleen and liver, these organs become engorged with blood. This can cause a rapid drop in hemoglobin to levels as low as 1-3g/dl. During sequestration episodes, the engorged organ(s) can be palpated during the abdominal exam. The risk for sequestration is greatest until age 3 years.

Sickle cells can cause infarcts (dead tissue due to lack of blood supply) in any area of the body including the lungs, spleen, bones, and brain. The resultant splenic infarcts are so numerous that the spleen eventually shrinks and becomes nonfunctional. This is called an autosplenectomy or functional asplenia because the body essentially caused the equivalent of removing a functional spleen. Autosplenectomy is complete by age 5 years. Brain infarcts cause strokes. Transient decrease in brain blood flow can also cause seizures.

Sickle cell disease is a common illness that affects millions of people worldwide. The populations that are most affected are those whose ancestors came from sub-Saharan Africa; Spanish-speaking regions in the Western Hemisphere (South America, Central America, and the Caribbean); Saudi Arabia; India; and Mediterranean countries such as Turkey, Greece, and Italy.

Approximately 100,000 Americans have sickle cell disease. SCD occurs among about 1 in every 365 African-American births and about 1 in 16,300 Hispanic-American births. About 1 in 13 African-American babies is born with sickle cell trait. Sickle cell trait helps prevent mortality due to malaria.

Newborn screening detects blood disorders such as sickle cell disease and approximately 40 genetic, developmental, and metabolic disorders. You may recall that when your child was first born, one of the final tests before discharge required 5 blood spots on a card, and you received a pink slip of paper. Your pediatrician used the number on your pink paper to obtain the results within the next 2 weeks. The newborn screening test only confirms that there is abnormal hemoglobin present. Another test called hemoglobin electrophoresis confirms the diagnosis.

There are different types of hemoglobin (Hb). The main types are Hemoglobin A, Hemoglobin S, Hemoglobin C, and Hemoglobin F. Hemoglobin A (HbA) is the most common type of hemoglobin in adults. Hemoglobin F (HbF) is found in the fetus (growing baby). Hemoglobin F holds onto oxygen more strongly than Hemoglobin A to facilitate the fetus getting the mother's oxygen. Once the baby is born, HbF levels gradually decrease as HbA levels increase. This change to HbA is usually complete by 1 year of age. Therefore, vaso-occlusive pain crises do not begin until around 6 months of age.

SCD has recessive gene inheritance. Both parents must contribute a Hemoglobin S (HbS) gene for SCD to occur. If one parent contributes a normal Hemoglobin A (HbA) gene and the other parent contributes a HbS gene, the child will have sickle cell trait. If both parents contribute a HbA gene, the child will have normal hemoglobin.

		Parent #1	
		HbA	HbS
Parent #2	HbA	AA Normal	AS Sickle Trait (carrier)
	HbS	SA Sickle Trait (carrier)	SS SCD Disease

25% chance of normal hemoglobin

50% chance of sickle cell trait

25% chance of sickle cell disease

Figure 1 – HbSS gene inheritance where both parents have sickle cell

**If one parent has HbSS and the other parent has sickle cell trait (HbAS), the chance of the child having SCD (HbSS) increases to 50%.

Hemoglobin SC disease is a hemoglobin disorder where one parent contributes a HbS gene and the other parent contributes a HbC gene. Hemoglobin SC patients get vaso-occlusive pain episodes, but far less frequently. Of note, there are other hemoglobin gene mutations called thalassemias.

Those with sickle cell trait live a relatively normal life as a carrier of the HbS gene. However, when the body is placed in extreme conditions, a vaso-occlusive pain episode may be triggered. Examples of these conditions are cold weather, wind, low humidity, lower oxygen levels in the air in high altitudes, dehydration, stress from extreme exercise in military boot camp or training for an athletic competition, and increased pressure in the atmosphere (e.g., while scuba diving). Alcohol and menses (the bleeding period of the menstrual cycle) can also trigger pain episodes.

Once the diagnosis is confirmed, the infant is referred to a specialist called a pediatric hematologist/oncologist (Peds Heme/Onc), who will direct all sickle cell related care until there is a transition to an adult hematologist. Your pediatrician should provide all general pediatric care such as physicals, immunizations, and sick visits unrelated to sickle cell or another specialty. Children with sickle cell disease are considered immunocompromised because their spleen is not functional. In addition to routine vaccinations, immunocompromised children are given additional doses of pneumococcal (the pneumonia vaccine) and meningococcal (the meningitis vaccine) vaccines on a special schedule. *Haemophilus influenzae* type b (Hib) is another bacterium that is normally destroyed by the spleen. Annual influenza (flu) vaccination is also strongly recommended because immunocompromised people are at a greater risk of having worse symptoms if infected.

If your child has been diagnosed with sickle cell disease, he or she should already have routine follow-up by Peds Heme/Onc. During every visit, hemoglobin levels are measured by obtaining a complete blood count (CBC). The normal hemoglobin level for a child ages 6-12 years is approximately 13.5g/dl but can vary with age, race, and sex. Weight, height, head circumference, and blood pressure should also be documented at every visit. A Transcranial

Doppler (ultrasound through the skull) is performed annually starting at 2 years of age to screen for risk of a stroke. Starting at age 10, children need annual dilated eye exams to check for retinopathy. Urine should also be tested annually to screen for kidney dysfunction.

Parents should receive education on how to manage their child's illness. This includes avoiding triggers like the cold or dehydration. Parents are also taught to palpate (feel) the spleen at least once a day when the child is healthy and more often when the child is sick. If a family member believes that the spleen is enlarged, the child should be taken for a medical evaluation immediately to confirm the increased size and obtain a CBC to determine whether a blood transfusion is necessary. Families should also be given a Fever Plan that should be enacted whenever the child has a temp above the stated threshold.

Parents should also be advised that children with sickle cell disease qualify for special needs services and school accommodations such as 504 programs. School notes should be provided to allow these children to drink fluids in class.

The main daily treatment for sickle cell disease is hydroxyurea. It is started between 6-9 months of age and is continued through adulthood. Hydroxyurea increases the amount of Hemoglobin F (fetal Hb). Higher amounts of HbF decrease the formation of HbS. This decreases the frequency and severity of vaso-occlusive pain episodes and decreases acute chest syndrome episodes. Since fewer sickle cells are produced, hemolytic anemia also occurs less frequently. Hydroxyurea has been shown to increase life expectancy. Folic acid may be recommended.

Penicillin VK (Pen VK) is another treatment. It is given as prophylaxis against bacteria that would normally be destroyed by the spleen. Prophylaxis is started by age 2 months and continued twice a day until the second pneumococcal polysaccharide vaccine (PPSV23) has been administered. The second PPSV23 vaccine is usually given between ages 5-7 years of age. Erythromycin is prescribed if your child has a penicillin allergy.

Blood transfusions are used to not only treat sickle cell disease but also to prevent complications from the illness. Transfusions are considered treatment when they are given to combat symptomatic anemia, acute chest syndrome, an acute stroke, and multiorgan failure. Symptomatic anemia is defined as when the body can no longer compensate for the decrease in hemoglobin. Your child may develop an increased heart rate, palpitations, hyperventilation, headache, lightheadedness, altered mental status (e.g., confusion, disorientation, agitation, inattention, change in behavior), paleness, cool and/or clammy skin, weakness, or fatigue. Transfusions are considered preventive when given to impede the development of a future stroke, acute chest syndrome episode, or recurrent priapism. Some children may be placed on a chronic transfusion regimen where they receive monthly blood transfusions or at least 8 transfusions per year. Chronic transfusions keep Hemoglobin

S below 30% of the total red blood cells. Chronic transfusions usually occur over a 6-month period.

There is a cure for sickle cell disease. The cure is stem cell transplantation. This treatment is recommended if there is a sibling donor match. Although curative, it is not recommended often because of the risk of sterility or even worse, death.

Pain medications are prescribed by your child's Peds Heme/Onc team and like other medications, are dosed by weight. Pain management care plans are individualized to the child. Acetaminophen and ibuprofen are prescribed for mild pain. For moderate to severe pain, children are prescribed opioids. Examples of opioids are morphine, Dilaudid (hydromorphone), Oxycontin (oxycodone), Lortab/Vicodin (hydrocodone + acetaminophen), and fentanyl. Fentanyl is the only medication that can be prescribed as a skin patch. Heating pads, massaging affected areas, and lots of fluids can be useful nonmedical treatments. Avoid ice or cold packs because cold is a trigger.

Should Maria go?

This is a trick question. No, Maria should not go to the urgent care center because she needs to go straight to the hospital for a medical evaluation and pain management.

Final Care Plan: When Maria arrived at the emergency room, she was in such severe pain that she was barely able to move and was lying on the table crying. Pain was reported as a 10 out of 10 on the pain scale. Maria was afebrile.

Heart rate was elevated due to pain. Oxygen saturation was 96% on room air. Her skin was pale and extremely jaundiced. Her sclerae (whites of the eyes) were also yellow. Maria's lungs were clear and she denied having any chest pain. Chest x-ray was negative. Maria was admitted for pain management and started on IV morphine. IV fluids were given for hydration. Although Maria did not require oxygen, it was still provided for comfort. Maria was discharged home once she could be switched back to oral pain medications.

Appendicitis

Zachary is an 11-year-old boy who started having severe sharp right lower quadrant (RLQ) pain over the past 6 hours. He has nausea and vomited twice. He has not eaten all day and is now unable to walk. No headache, ear pain, or sore throat. No diarrhea or pain with urination. What is the diagnosis?

Zachary has appendicitis. The appendix is a small pouch located at the start of the large intestine. Appendicitis is inflammation of the appendix. If the appendix is not removed in time, it can perforate (burst).

The most common symptoms of appendicitis are RLQ tenderness, difficulty walking, loss of appetite, pain with jumping, nausea, vomiting, and fever. Abdominal pain and vomiting are present at all ages. Starting at the age of 5, children can discern that the right lower quadrant is most tender to touch. Pain migration from the periumbilical (near the belly button) region to the RLQ is more likely to present in children ages 12 years and older. Involuntary guarding (i.e., tensing and moving away when touched) and rebound tenderness (i.e., pain after pressing on the abdomen) are signs of bowel perforation. When there is a concern for appendicitis, your child will be instructed to have nothing to eat or drink (NPO) because the stomach should be clear during the surgery to prevent vomiting and possible aspiration (i.e., vomited food getting into the lungs) during the procedure. Morphine is given for pain management and antibiotics are given to prevent infection. Both are given intravenously (via IV).

Ultrasound, CT scan, and MRI are imaging modalities used to diagnose appendicitis. Ultrasound does not require radiation, but the accuracy depends on the person performing the test. CT scan of the abdomen is more accurate than ultrasound, but a CT scan equals at least 100 x-rays. An advantage of a CT scan is that the scan takes minutes. If your child needs an abdominal CT scan, the images may be enhanced using IV contrast to light up the blood vessels. Some institutions may also administer oral contrast to light up the digestive system. Many patients have difficulty tolerating oral contrast due to its taste and the large volume. MRI abdomen is as accurate as a CT scan and does not use radiation but may not be available at every hospital. Also, the procedure is very loud (patients wear headphones) and takes at least 30-60 minutes. Younger children have difficulty lying still for that amount of time and require sedation. Most facilities will start with an ultrasound and move on to CT scan or MRI if ultrasound results are unclear.

Once the diagnosis is confirmed, the appendix is removed in a procedure called an appendectomy. An appendectomy can be laparoscopic (i.e., removal via small incisions using a camera and long arm tools) or open (i.e., a long incision down the abdomen to have an open visualization).

Should Zachary go?

Yes. Zachary needs to have a full abdominal exam. I have seen cases of severe abdominal pain that were due to constipation or gas.

Final Care Plan: Zachary had a temp of 100.4° and was lying still. He had RLQ tenderness and collapsed in pain when he attempted to jump. He was transferred to the ER where an MRI showed appendicitis. He underwent an appendectomy and is now doing well.

Urinary Tract Infection (UTI)

Rachel is a 5-year-old girl who has been having burning with urination, lower abdominal pain, and has been urinating more frequently than usual over the past 2 days. Her mother also notes that Rachel has been unable to make it to the bathroom in time. Rachel has been potty trained since the age of two. No fever, lower back pain, or vomiting. When asked to demonstrate how she wipes after using the bathroom, she does a back-to-front motion. Why is Rachel having these symptoms?

Rachel has a urinary tract infection (UTI). The urinary tract includes the kidneys, ureters, bladder, and urethra. Cystitis is an infection of the bladder and is the most common type of UTI. When the UTI spreads to the ureters and kidneys, it is called pyelonephritis. Fever, flank pain (pain over the kidneys), and vomiting are symptoms that would make one suspicious of pyelonephritis.

Viruses can also cause UTIs, but the most common causes are *E. coli* and other bacteria found in the stool. UTIs are more commonly seen in girls than boys. One possible reason is that the female urethra is shorter, which creates a shorter distance for bacteria to reach the bladder. Wiping in a back-to-front motion can facilitate bringing bacteria from the stool forward to the urethra. Uncircumcised males are at an increased risk of contracting a UTI than circumcised males.

When there is suspicion of a UTI, it is best to obtain a urine specimen before starting antibiotics. Antibiotics can cause falsely negative results because they partially treated the infection. Also, obtaining a urine specimen can help guide antibiotic treatment so that we know exactly which bacteria we are treating, and which antibiotic is the best choice. This avoids jumping unknowingly from antibiotic to antibiotic. Antibiotics may be started prior to receiving urine results depending on the severity of symptoms. Omnicef (cefdinir), Bactrim (trimethoprim & sulfamethoxazole), and Macrobid/Macrodantin (nitrofurantoin) are commonly used antibiotics in children.

The first step in obtaining a urine culture is cleaning the skin, which limits possible urine contamination by either normal bacteria that live on the skin or bacteria from a previous stool that came from the back to the front. Betadine is a brownish fluid that is commonly used to clean the skin when a sterile field is necessary. You may also see pre-packaged applicator sponges that release a clear fluid called chlorhexidine. Once the area is deemed sterile, the urine is collected.

The most accurate method to obtain a urine specimen is via suprapubic aspiration, which is when a sterile needle is inserted into the skin of the lower abdomen until it reaches the bladder. Urine is extracted via the needle and placed in a sterile container. This method is the most accurate because it is easier to thoroughly clean the flat surface of the abdomen vs the skin in the genital region. This method, however, is painful and only used when necessary.

The second most accurate method is urinary catheterization. During this procedure, a small tube is inserted into the urethra until it reaches the bladder. This tube is the size of a feeding tube that is inserted into the nose. The tube is connected to a sterile syringe that can be drawn back to collect urine, which is then transferred to a sterile container. This method is normally used when a patient is incontinent (i.e., not potty trained). It is an uncomfortable procedure, but the tube is very small and only in place temporarily unlike when a larger Foley catheter is placed to measure urine over time.

The third most accurate technique is the clean-catch method. A clean catch specimen is obtained when a sterile container is held under the outer opening of the urethra for urine collection. This is most easily achieved when a person has urinary continence (i.e., potty-trained). The advantage of this tactic is that it is noninvasive and therefore pain-free.

Parents occasionally ask about using a urine bag for collection. The urine bag has adhesive and is attached to the skin surrounding the urethra. The issue with bagging is that this method is not sterile, which increases the risk for cross contamination. The only way a bagged specimen can be deemed acceptable is if the urine culture is completely negative. If a bagged specimen is positive, it should be confirmed with a sterile specimen. As a result, I do not recommend bagged urine specimens.

Next, the urine is tested. A urinalysis (UA) is a screening test for urine. Abnormal UA results are confirmed with a urine culture. A urine culture shows whether there is bacterial growth and the antibiotics that can be used to treat the infection (sensitivity).

A negative urine culture result means that there was not a significant growth of bacteria. If antibiotics were started preemptively, they would then be stopped. A viral UTI will yield a negative urine culture. Viral UTIs resolve on their own.

If the urine culture is positive, the antibiotic given will be checked to see if it was a good choice. If the bacteria is sensitive to the antibiotic, the antibiotic will be continued for completion of the prescribed duration, which is usually for a total of 7-10 days. Ciprofloxacin is an antibiotic given to older teens and adults and in uncomplicated cases, its duration is a 3-day course.

Should Rachel go?

Yes. Rachel should provide a urine specimen for testing prior to starting antibiotics.

Final Care Plan: Rachel was prescribed cefdinir pending her urine culture results. The urine culture grew *E. coli*, which was sensitive to cefdinir. When Rachel's family was called with lab results 3 days later, Rachel's pain had resolved. Her parents were advised to complete the antibiotic course and follow up with her pediatrician for repeat urine testing once the antibiotic course was complete.

Testicular Torsion

George is a 13-year-old boy who has been complaining of sharp left testicular pain for the past 3 hours. He reports that he was playing video games and the testicular pain began suddenly upon standing. The pain is constant and does not radiate. He rated the pain a 10 out 10 on the pain scale. Since the pain began, George has been complaining of nausea and he vomited once. He denies any trauma to the area. No pain with urination. What is the cause of George's pain?

George has testicular torsion. Boys usually have two testicles that sit in the scrotum (sac). Each testicle hangs from a cord called the spermatic cord. This cord contains the vas deferens (the duct that the sperm travels through when it leaves the testicle), blood vessels, and nerves. Testicular torsion occurs when the testicle twists on its spermatic cord. This is a medical emergency because the blood supply, and more importantly, the oxygen gets cut off when the testicle gets torsed.

If the torsion is not corrected quickly, the testicle could die. A testicle has 97-100% viability (i.e., ability to survive) if the testicle is detorsed within 4-6 hours. After 12 hours, keeping the testicle alive decreases to 20-61% viability. After 24 hours, there is a 0-24% viability.

The primary symptom of testicular torsion is sudden, severe testicular pain, usually on one side. Other symptoms are a scrotal sac that is red, tender, and swollen; an enlarged testicle; nausea; vomiting; and lower abdominal pain. When available, Doppler ultrasound (i.e., ultrasound of the blood vessels that checks for blood flow) determines whether the cause is testicular torsion. Once the diagnosis is confirmed, your child will need a urologist to perform a surgery called an orchiopexy. After the detorsion is complete, the urologist tacks the testicle in place to prevent torsion from occurring again. Occasionally, the urologist will tack down the other testicle as a preventative measure.

Should George go?

No, George should not go to an urgent care center because he will automatically be sent to the emergency room for a Doppler ultrasound. Please do not waste your time. The timer is ticking!

Final Care Plan: Upon arriving in the ER, George was in severe pain. His left testicle was enlarged and the scrotum was red and tender. Doppler ultrasound confirmed the torsion. Urology brought him to the OR for emergency surgery. The testicle was still viable after the orchiopexy.

Pediculosis Capitis (Lice)

Charlotte is a 9-year-old girl who has been constantly scratching her scalp for the past week. There is a flat, red rash at the nape of her neck. No other rash is noted on the body. No hair loss. Charlotte's mother noticed tiny, white spots on her daughter's hair, but the scalp is not dry or flaky. The spots are not easily removable when her mother attempts to brush her hair. Charlotte does not have a history of dandruff or eczema. No new shampoo. Charlotte returned from overnight summer camp 8 days ago and admits that she borrowed a bunk mate's comb after misplacing hers. Why is Charlotte's scalp so itchy?

Charlotte has Pediculosis capitis, a condition caused by an infestation of the hair and scalp by a parasite called *Pediculus humanus capitis. The layman's term for the parasite is* the head louse. Head lice are normally found on the scalp, hence the name. Pediculosis capitis occurs worldwide and is seen in all socioeconomic backgrounds. Children are affected more than adults. Girls are affected more than boys. In the United States, white children are affected much more frequently than African-American children. One proposed theory as to why there is a lower incidence in American-American children is that it is more difficult for head lice to grasp the shape or width of certain hair types with their legs.

A female adult head louse can lay 7-10 eggs per day. These eggs aka nits are very sticky and get firmly attached to the hair shaft. Nits can be confused with dandruff, but dandruff can be easily removed from the hair. The nits hatch in 8 days and release nymphs that take another 8 days to mature into adult lice. Adult lice are gray-white and approximately 2-3 millimeters in length. They feed on the scalp and adjacent areas of the face and neck including behind the ears. They are rarely found on the eyebrows and eyelashes. Adult lice can live for about 1 month on the scalp, but can only survive up to 55 hours if they fall off a host and are unable to feed. Lice cannot jump or fly. They get primarily transferred by direct head-to-head contact of an infested person to another person. Rarely, head lice can also be spread by sharing clothing, combs, hair accessories, brushes, towels, stuffed animals, or lying on a bed or couch that has recently been in contact with an infested person.

The main symptom of lice infestation is itching. The lice saliva that is injected during feeding causes an allergic reaction. This reaction is not immediate unless your child has been sensitized by a previous infestation. If this is the first infestation, sensitization may take 4-6 weeks before the itching begins. Your child may also complain of a tickling feeling or something moving in his or her hair. Scratch marks may be visible on the scalp, neck, and behind the ears. Your child may have difficulty sleeping because head lice are most active in the dark. Due to the lack of sleep, they may be easily annoyed.

Diagnosis is made by visualizing live lice, but lice are difficult to see because they move quickly and avoid light.

If lice are not seen, it is still likely that your child has lice if nits are found within ¼ inch from the base of hair shafts. Nits that are found further than ¼ inch from the scalp are almost always dead or already hatched. If the only nits that are seen are further than ¼ inch and no live lice are visualized, the infestation is probably old and does not need to be treated. The best way to perform a lice check is by carefully parting and combing through your child's entire head twice using a fine-toothed nit comb. If you do not have a nit comb readily available, you can use a regular fine-toothed comb, but be aware that the teeth in a nit comb are more closely together to facilitate combing out lice.

First line treatment for head lice is the use of medicated shampoos, cream rinses, and lotions called Nix (permethrin 1% lotion) or Rid (pyrethrin). These topical treatments kill lice but do not kill nits. Prescription formulations are more difficult to find so over-the-counter options are suggested first. Be sure to follow the head lice directions for each medication exactly as written. If your community has head lice that are resistant to these medications, other options like Ovide (malathion) may be used. Malathion kills lice and nits.

We will include the Nix 1% Crème rinse instructions as an example. Wash hair with a non-conditioning shampoo, rinse with water, and towel dry hair. Hair will still be damp. Next, apply a sufficient volume of permethrin solution/rinse to saturate the hair and scalp. Also apply behind the ears and at the base of the neck. Leave on hair for 10 minutes before rinsing off with warm water. Remove remaining nits with the nit comb that was included in the box. Repeat in 7 to 10 days if live lice or nits are observed. The optimal time to repeat is on Day 9 based on the life cycle of head lice.

Topical Application Tips

1. Use gloves when applying medicine.

2. Always rinse the medicine off over a sink. Rinsing the medicine during a shower or bath will lead to it running off the head onto the rest of the body.

3. Use warm water instead of hot water.

4. Avoid the eyes during this process. You may place a towel over your child's eyes as an extra measure.

5. Never place a plastic bag on your child's head.

6. Do not leave your child alone with medicine in his or her hair.

7. Store medicine out of sight and reach of children.

Another treatment option is manual removal with a nit comb without any topical medicines. This option is extremely tedious. There are professional head lice treatment facilities around the country. Many are known as "The Lice Lady" of their area.

Household Recommendations

Wash the clothing and linen used during the 2 days prior to treatment in hot water and dry the items on a high-heat setting. Items that cannot be washed may be dry-cleaned or stored in a sealed plastic bag for 2 weeks. Vacuuming the furniture and carpeting that your child sat or laid on may be beneficial although the risk of transmission from these sites is low. Household members should be examined and treated if live lice or nits within ¼ inch of the scalp are detected. Automatically treat any household members including yourself who share a bed with your child.

Return To School

Medically speaking, your child does not need to be excluded from school due to the presence of lice or nits. However, some schools have a "no-nit" policy and do not allow students to return to school while nits are still seen.

Should Charlotte go?

No. Her mother visualized several nits cemented in place within ¼ inch of the base of the hair shafts. No live lice were seen. The recommendation is a topical OTC lice medicine.

Final Care Plan: Charlotte's mother used Nix Crème Rinse. On Day 7, the only nits visualized were greater than ¼ inch from the base of the hair shafts. No live lice were seen. She did not require a second treatment.

Scabies

Aaron is a 14-year-old boy who is complaining of intense itchiness of the hands, armpits, belly button, and waist for the past 4 days. There are small, red bumps in those areas. He also noticed that there are small, red lines in between his fingers. The rash is not crusting. No fever. No new foods, clothing, medications, soaps, detergents, lotions, or new pet exposures. He denies being in any wooded or bushy areas. He returned home from boarding school for summer vacation 2 weeks ago. Parents were notified that his dorm mates have similar symptoms. What is the cause of Aaron's rash?

Aaron has scabies. Scabies is an infestation of the skin of a parasite called *Sarcoptes scabiei. I*t is an 8-legged whitish-brown mite. Female mites measure approximately 0.4 by 0.3 mm. Male mites are slightly larger than half that size and are rarely seen. Adult mites do not have eyes. Male mites create temporary shallow pits in the skin to feed and remain until they find a female to mate. After mating, female mites burrow into the epidermis (i.e., the top layer of skin) by secreting an enzyme that causes damage to the skin cells. Female mites continue to extend the burrow and lay 2-3 eggs per day until their death 4-6 weeks later. Larvae hatch in 3-4 days. Mites can survive 24-36 hours without a host at room temperature in average humidity but can survive longer in colder conditions with higher humidity. During an initial infestation, only approximately

10-15 mites are present. During subsequent infestations, half that number appears. They get transferred by direct and prolonged skin-to-skin contact from an infested person to another person. Casual skin contact and transfer from clothing or bedding or unlikely.

Scabies is a common infestation, affecting 100 million people worldwide. It can affect individuals of all ages and socioeconomic backgrounds. Crowded conditions increase the risk for scabies infestations. Epidemics can occur in institutional settings such as long-term care facilities.

Classic scabies presents as a widespread intensely itchy rash with a characteristic distribution. The tiny red bumps are often in short straight or wavy lines. The bumps are the sites where the mites burrowed into the skin. They are most commonly seen on the wrists and hands, especially on the side in the webbing between the fingers. Other locations are the armpits, breast areolae, belly button, waist, male groin, behind the elbows, and on the ankles. Scalp involvement may be seen in younger children. Similar to head lice, itchiness is the result of a delayed allergic reaction. A primary sensitivity develops 3-6 weeks after exposure to the mite, mite feces, and mite eggs. In previously infested patients, symptoms usually begin within 1-3 days after infestation.

The diagnosis of scabies is confirmed through the detection of scabies mites, eggs, or feces with microscopic examination. However, since there are so few mites present during an infestation, it is difficult to find these things on exam. A presumptive diagnosis is sometimes made based upon a consistent history and physical examination.

Scabies is treated with the same medicines as head lice, but the concentrations and instructions are different. Elimite (permethrin) cream is a 5% strength to treat scabies. The application instructions dictate that the cream should be massaged thoroughly into the skin from the neck to the bottom of the feet including under the fingernails and toenails. Since scabies can affect the scalp of infants, the cream should be applied from the top of the head (sparing the eyes and mouth) to the bottom of the feet for this population. The cream should be left on for 8-14 hours before removing it in a shower or bath. Repeat application if living mites are observed 14 days after treatment. One application is usually curative.

Should Aaron go?

Yes. Most people are not familiar with the signs and symptoms of scabies to recognize an infestation. Also, since treatment involves applying cream all over the body, your child should be evaluated first.

Final Care Plan: On exam, Aaron had small red bumps on his fingers, wrists, armpits, and on his waist. Burrows were appreciated on the webbing in between his fingers and on his wrists. He denied any itchiness of the face and scalp. Aaron's father was advised to assist in applying permethrin 5% cream from the neck to the soles of the feet. The cream was left on overnight for 10 hours and rinsed off in the morning. Aaron did not require a second treatment.

Enterobiasis (Pinworms)

Quinn is a 5-year-old girl who has been constantly digging inside her pants for the past 3 days. She is scratching in the front and the back. Quinn is potty trained, but still has a parent or teacher wipe her after passing stool. No burning with urination. There is no rash in the groin or near the anus. No stool or toilet tissue stuck between her cheeks. No abdominal pain, vomiting, or diarrhea. She has been having difficulty sleeping for the past 2 nights. Quinn plays in the sandbox at her school. What is wrong with Quinn?

Quinn has enterobiasis aka pinworms. Enterobiasis is an infestation by a parasite called *Enterobius vermicularis.* It is the most common worm infection in the United States and Western Europe. Forty million Americans have pinworms. Infection occurs in all socioeconomic groups, most frequently in children ages 5-10 years. Transmission rates increase when people live in closed, crowded conditions.

Transmission occurs primarily via the fecal-oral route. This is when a small amount of stool inadvertently gets ingested by mouth. Often, an infected child scratches himself, picks up an egg, and then transfers the egg to the sandbox or a toilet seat where another child unknowingly picks it up and later transfers it to his mouth with a contaminated hand. Other person-to-person transmission possibilities are when a person eats food touched by contaminated hands or a person handles contaminated clothes or bed linens. Infection may also occur via contact transmission when a person touches a surface like curtains or carpeting that is contaminated with eggs. In addition, eggs can become airborne, get inhaled, and swallowed. transmission. The egg is swallowed and travels to the small intestines where it hatches.

Once the egg is swallowed, it travels to the small intestine where it hatches, and a larva is produced. Adult worms mainly live in the small intestine near the appendix. Adult worms are whitish-gray and threadlike, measuring between ¼ - ½ inch long. When a female adult worm gets pregnant, she travels through the rest of the intestines and outside of the body where she deposits her eggs within the skin folds around the anus. The female adult worm tends to emerge overnight approximately 2-3 hours after the infected person fell asleep.

Itching occurs because the presence of the worms and eggs on the skin causes an inflammatory reaction. Itchiness can be so intense that an infected person scratches to the point of leaving marks. Deep scratches need to be monitored because they can get infected by bacteria. In addition to perianal itching, girls may also have itching in the vulvar region (i.e., outer area of the female genitals) if the worms migrate to other sites including the vulva, vagina (birth canal), and urethra.

Re-infection can occur when an infected person scratches, an egg gets lodged beneath the fingernails, and swallows it, thus restarting the entire cycle. This is called autoinfection. The eggs can also be transferred from underneath the fingernails to another person. The timespan from swallowing infective eggs to the laying of new eggs by adult female worms takes approximately 1 month. Each female worm can produce at least 10,000 eggs. Adult worms live for 2-3 months. Most pinworm infestations produce hundreds of adult worms. It takes 4-6 hours for the deposited eggs to mature into infective eggs with larvae inside. The eggs start to become less infective after 1-2 days under warm and dry conditions but may survive more than 2 weeks in cooler, more humid environments.

Diagnosis is made in one of three ways: 1) whitish worms are visible in the perianal region or on the undergarments, 2) the Paddle test aka Scotch-tape test is positive, or 3) samples collected from beneath the fingernails have eggs. The Paddle test is performed by either pressing a plastic paddle coated with a sticky surface or a piece of Scotch tape against the perianal region onto a glass slide, which is then examined under a microscope. The best results are when the test is performed at night or immediately after awakening prior to hatching. Stool studies are not useful because the eggs are deposited outside of the body.

Pinworms are treated with oral anthelmintic (anti-worm) medications like pyrantel pamoate/Reese Pinworm medicine, mebendazole, or albendazole. Reese Pinworm is available without prescription as a two-dose treatment. The first dose is given on Day 1. The second dose is given on Day 14 to prevent possible reinfection. In cases of confirmed enterobiasis, the entire household should be treated regardless of their symptoms. All bedding and clothing should be washed. Clipping fingernails and frequent handwashing help reduce reinfection and spread of infection to others. Showering is preferred over taking a bath because bathwater could become infected with pinworm eggs.

Should Quinn go?

No. The history of the perianal and vulvar itching without a rash or any other explainable cause is sufficient to make a clinical diagnosis.

Final Care Plan: Quinn was given the two doses of Reese Pinworm Medicine. Itchiness resolved.

Tick Bite/Is It Lyme Disease?

Paula is a 7-year-old girl with a tick on her upper back. Paula's mother noticed it when she did her nightly tick check. Paula lives near a wooded area and plays outside whenever weather permits. No fever or rash. Paula does not have any pets. Why is Paula's mother so concerned?

Paula's mother is concerned about Lyme disease. Lyme disease is a tick-borne illness caused by a bacterium called *Borrelia burgdorferi*. Ticks need to feed for 36-48 hours to transmit the infection.

The medical term for the bull's-eye or target-like rash is erythema migrans. Erythema migrans usually appears 7-14 days after the tick bite and is seen near the bite site. Unfortunately, many tick bites go unnoticed, and if the tick bite occurs in an obscure area like the scalp, the rash may not be seen. A bull's-eye is seen because the rash has a red center, an outer ring of clearing, and another ring of redness. The rash is flat, does not have a scale, and must measure at least 5 cm in diameter. Other symptoms that are seen while erythema migrans is present include fatigue, fever, headache, neck pain, joint pain, and muscle aches.

If Lyme disease goes untreated, the symptoms progress to arthritis (joint inflammation), Bell's Palsy (1 sided facial paralysis), meningitis (inflammation of the layers around the brain and spinal cord), and inflammation of the heart muscle that can cause an arrhythmia.

If you want to test your child for Lyme titers, you should wait at least 2 weeks for antibodies to be created.

There are scenarios where prophylactic antibiotics are recommended. The tick needs to be identified as a deer tick (dog ticks do not cause Lyme), the tick needs to be attached for at least 36 hours, prophylaxis is given within 72 hours of tick removal, the bite occurs in a highly endemic area (Northeast & Mid Atlantic US, Minnesota, and Wisconsin), and doxycycline can be used. Prophylaxis treatment is a single dose of doxycycline.

If your child is diagnosed with Lyme disease and older than 8 years old, the treatment of choice is a 10-day course of doxycycline. If your child is younger than age 8 or is allergic to doxycycline, acceptable alternatives are a 14-day course of amoxicillin or cefuroxime (Ceftin).

You can try to prevent tick bites by using DEET insect repellent, wearing sleeves and long pants when in wooded areas, and performing a tick check once a day. Ticks can be removed at home by using sharp tweezers and grabbing the tick's head as close to the person's skin as possible. Pull the tick straight out.

Should Paula go?

Maybe. If Paula's parents are unable to remove the tick, Paula should be seen for tick removal.

Final Care Plan: Paula's parents did not want to touch the tick. Paula was taken to an urgent care center where the tick was removed during evaluation. The rest of the exam was normal. No rash was seen. Since Paula's mother performs a tick check every night, it is unlikely that the tick has been feeding for over 24 hours, especially since the area is easy to see. Antibiotic prophylaxis was not given.

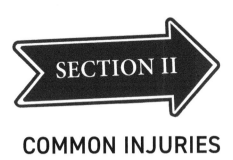

COMMON INJURIES

Concussion/Head Injury

Harry is a ten-year-old boy who fell backward and hit his head while playing soccer 30 minutes ago. He did not lose consciousness and remembers everything. He stayed on the sideline for the remainder of soccer practice. When he got home, his mother applied ice to the area. He complained of a headache. No other symptoms. Does Harry have a concussion?

A concussion is a head injury that results from a direct blow to the head, face, neck, or anywhere else in the body where the head has an acceleration/deceleration jostling of the brain inside the skull that causes a set of prolonged symptoms. These symptoms can last days to weeks to months. Every injury is different. You cannot predict how long symptoms will last. You can only track improvement or worsening of symptoms.

Signs and symptoms of concussion include loss of consciousness, memory loss, confusion, dizziness, blurry vision, diplopia (i.e., seeing double), light sensitivity, noise sensitivity, tinnitus (i.e., ringing in his ears), staggering balance, weakness of one arm or leg, nausea, vomiting more than once, decreased alertness when awake, inconsolability, change in behavior, and seizures. Loss of consciousness is not necessary for a concussion diagnosis to be made.

Many parents ask about pupil size. You do not need to take out a ruler. If the pupil size is unequal, it is very apparent. One pupil will be dilated (larger than usual). Also, by the time there is a change in pupil size, your child will already be vomiting.

Your child is allowed to vomit once. If your child vomits more than once, go to the emergency room for evaluation. Other symptoms that warrant immediate attention are staggering balance, weakness of one arm or leg, nausea, vomiting more than once, decreased alertness when awake, inconsolability, change in behavior, and seizures.

When a person sustains a head injury, the main concern is that the injury caused an intracranial hemorrhage (bleeding in the brain). Most people will start exhibiting the concerning signs of an intracranial hemorrhage within two hours after injury. If your child is being evaluated for a possible concussion, you may have to stay in the facility for at least two hours for observation. During your child's medical evaluation, the entire body should be checked for any injuries not previously disclosed. The head should be examined for any skull depressions or scalp hematomas to clinically rule out a skull fracture. Your child should also have a complete neurological exam that includes checking pupils, reflexes, strength, memory, and ability to complete certain movements. If the exam remains normal, your child is allowed to go home, but you should continue to monitor your child closely for the next 24 hours.

Your child is allowed to go to sleep. If you keep your child awake, this could cause irritability from your child becoming overtired. Set your alarm to check on your child twice overnight. Your child should be sleeping comfortably.

If your child is having difficulty breathing or a fitful sleep where he or she tosses more than usual, go to the emergency room.

It is expected that your child should have a headache after a head injury. Acetaminophen can be given every 4 hours as needed for pain. Avoid ibuprofen for the first 24 hours! Ibuprofen can thin the blood. It is recommended that stimulation be reduced if possible. You can help reduce stimulation of your child by keeping him or her in a dim room, limiting screen time (e.g., TV, video games, texting, tablet, etc.). We do not want to exacerbate any possible brain bleed. A severe headache that does not subside 4-6 hours after injury warrants immediate

Reduce stimulation by keeping patient in a dimly lit room and limiting screen time (TV, video games, texting, tablet, etc.). If your child is diagnosed with a concussion, it is helpful to give frequent breaks when studying. Your child may be able to tolerate attending school but should be allowed to put his or her head on the desk to rest whenever necessary.

There is no longer a set period of time that your child has to rest prior to returning to play. Returning to full activity depends on how quickly your child returns to baseline. It is recommended that follow-up with your pediatrician should occur 2-3 days after the head injury because this is the period where the symptoms peak and will be at their worst. If the symptoms have resolved, your child can be started on a stepwise return to play. If symptoms still persist, your child will have serial follow-ups with the pediatrician for reevaluations until the concussion resolves.

Should Harry go?

Yes. As stated above, Harry needs to have a comprehensive physical exam that includes a complete neurological exam.

Final Care Plan: On exam, Harry had point tenderness over the area where he hit his head. There was a flat, reddish bruise, but no scalp swelling or bony depressions. The neurological exam was normal. Harry was given acetaminophen for pain. He was observed for 1 hour and there were no changes noted on the discharge exam. Based on the history of events and the normal neurological exam, Harry did not meet the criteria for a concussion. He continued acetaminophen as needed for the next 24 hours. He also continued the ice packs for the next 48 hours, which helped the swelling. Harry followed up with his pediatrician in 2 days and had a normal exam. He was cleared to return to the gym without restriction.

Corneal Abrasion

Tiffany is an 8-year-old girl who suddenly started complaining of right eye pain after she was poked in the eye by her baby sister. She was holding her sister, who was touching her face when the baby playfully hit her. Tiffany is now tearing and is unable to open the right eye due to pain. She keeps complaining that it feels like she has something in her eye. No bleeding was seen. Why is Tiffany unable to open her eye?

Tiffany has a corneal abrasion. The cornea is the outer transparent layer that covers the iris (i.e., the pigmented portion of the eye) and the pupil (i.e., the dark center of the eye). A corneal abrasion is a common superficial eye injury due to eye trauma, foreign body, or contact lens. Corneal abrasions are painful. People complain of a foreign body sensation even if no foreign body is present. They are sensitive to light and keep that eye closed. Vision is usually unaffected unless the abrasion is large and goes over the area that covers the pupil.

Corneal abrasions are visualized by performing a fluorescein test. Fluorescein is a fluorescent dye that coats the eye. To perform the test, an anesthetic eye drop like tetracaine is placed into the eye first to relieve the pain so that your child's eye can easily open. One to two drops of fluorescein are placed in the affected eye to coat the eyeball. Some fluorescein drops come in combination with an anesthetic; tetracaine is not used with these formulations.

Fluorescein is irritating to the eye. Many people report that their eyes burned for almost 30 seconds after the drop was administered. They are advised to keep their eye closed until the pain resolves.

Once the eye is opened, the examiner turns off the overhead light and turns on an instrument called a Woods light. The Woods light emits black light. The fluorescein fills the space within the abrasion, causing the shape of the abrasion to be seen. If a corneal abrasion is visualized, a vision screen is performed to determine if there are any changes in the visual acuity (how well the patient can see where 20/20 is normal vision). If the vision screen is normal, your child can be discharged home and started an antibiotic eye drop or ointment to prevent infection. These antibiotics are the same as the ones used to treat conjunctivitis (pink eye). Acetaminophen or ibuprofen can be used to treat the pain. Warm washcloth compresses 5 minutes on and 5 minutes off can also provide comfort. Pain usually resolves by the following morning. If your child is still complaining of eye pain the following day, he or she needs to be seen by an ophthalmologist or optometrist.

Should Tiffany go?

Yes. She needs an eye exam that includes a fluorescein test.

Final Care Plan: On exam, Tiffany's eye was tearing and slightly red. No foreign body was seen. The eyelids were normal. The fluorescein test visualized one small corneal abrasion. The vision screen was normal. Tiffany was discharged home on a 3-day course of erythromycin eye ointment.

Radial Head Subluxation (Nursemaid's Elbow/ Elbow Dislocation)

Fiona is a 4-year-old girl who stopped moving her left arm 2 hours ago. Her father was swinging her around by her left arm when she stumbled forward. Fiona's father pulled her arm upward to prevent her from falling. She screamed and started crying immediately afterward. She did not hit her elbow or wrist. No swelling was seen. Fiona is no longer crying, but she is only using her right hand to practice the piano. Fiona has never had a similar injury. What happened to Fiona's arm?

Fiona has a nursemaid's elbow. Nursemaid's elbow is an elbow injury where the radius (one of the forearm bones) gets dislocated after being pulled. The medical term is a radial head subluxation. The injury is referred to as a nursemaid's elbow to historically describe a maid pulling a child along while walking down the street. Dislocation occurs because the ligaments are looser when children are under the age of 5 years. It can occur through ages up to 6-7 years, but it typically occurs between the ages of 1-4 years. Approximately 20,000 American children get this injury every year. It occurs more in girls than in boys and the left arm gets injured more often than the right arm.

The mechanism of injury is usually a pulling or twisting of the forearm while holding onto the wrist or hand. Parents often report that they were swinging or lifting their children by their arms. Male caregivers tend to report that they were play-wrestling with their children. Female care-givers tend to report that their child pulled away, tripped, or suddenly started crying while getting dressed.

Nursemaid's elbow is painful, but the area is not ten-der to touch. The bones do not look deformed. There is no bruising or swelling. Your child will avoid moving the injured arm. The elbow will either be extended straight out, or it will be slightly bent and held with the forearm pronat-ed (i.e., forearm position where the palm is facing down).

Imaging is usually unnecessary if the story is the clas-sic presentation of a pull injury in a child under the age of 5 and the exam does not show signs of a fracture such as tenderness to the area, swelling, bruising, or a deformity of the arm. If any of these symptoms are present and the child fell onto the arm, x-rays should be performed to rule out fracture prior to manipulating the arm.

Once a nursemaid's elbow diagnosis is confirmed, the dislocated elbow is reduced (i.e., put back in its original place). Reduction can be performed using two methods.

The preferred method is the hyperpronation meth-od. During this method, the person performing the pro-cedure will grip your child's left wrist with one hand and your child's elbow with the other hand. The forearm is then hyperpronated (i.e., twisted in a position where the palm turns downward in a circular motion and goes past being parallel to the floor). The reduction is successful if a click is felt and/or heard by the person holding the elbow. The "click" is the head of the radius popping back into place.

This method is taught to parents whose children repeatedly dislocate their elbows so they can be reduced at home as long as the history is consistent with a nursemaid's elbow injury.

The other method is called the hypersupination method. During this method, your child's forearm is twisted in a position where the palm is turned upwards in a circular motion and goes past being parallel to the floor until the radius clicks back into place.

Your child will likely scream and cry at the moment that the elbow is reduced, but the pain usually resolves within 5-10 minutes. Your child may still avoid using the arm after a successful reduction out of fear that moving it will cause pain. Do not try to move your child's arm. Let your child play or provide a distraction for a few minutes. Afterward, encourage your child to reach upward to grab a toy or lollipop. Another trick is to have your child give a High Five. The longer that the elbow was dislocated, the longer it may take for the pain to resolve. For example, if the elbow were dislocated for several hours, your child may not move the arm for the rest of the night. You may give your child a dose of acetaminophen or ibuprofen for the pain. If your child still refuses to move the arm by the following morning, the elbow should be reevaluated. X-rays will likely be performed at that time.

Should Fiona go?

Yes. This is the first time that she has dislocated her elbow. A history should be taken to ensure that the mechanism of injury is consistent with a nursemaid's elbow. The entire extremity should be examined from the clavicle (collarbone) down to the hand to rule out any other injuries.

Final Care Plan: There was no tenderness on exam. Pulses were normal. Fiona's elbow was reduced using the hyperpronation method (turning the palm down). She started moving the arm 5 minutes later and reported that her pain had completely resolved. To prevent this injury in the future, parents were advised to hold Fiona by the upper arm or elbow when they are walking together instead of pulling her by the hand. Also, lift Fiona by the upper arms or under her arms when picking her up.

Supracondylar Fracture (Fracture of the Humerus)

Jared is a 7-year-old boy who has had right elbow pain, bruising, and swelling since this afternoon. The upper part of the elbow no longer looks straight and is clearly deformed. While at the park, he slipped from the monkey bars and fell onto his elbow. He was brought back home where ice was applied to the elbow. He was given a dose of ibuprofen for the pain. He cannot move his arm. What kind of injury does Jared have?

Jared has a supracondylar fracture. Fracture is the medical term for a break in the bone. A supracondylar fracture is a fracture of the lower end of the humerus in the elbow region. The humerus is the bone between the shoulder and the elbow. A common cause of this injury is when a child falls onto his or her outstretched arm and the elbow gets hyperextended (i.e., straightened past the point of normal).

A medical evaluation should be performed immediately to not only look for any other bony injuries but to complete a neurovascular examination. Neurovascular exams check for any nerve damage or abnormal pulses. Pain medication should be prior to obtaining an elbow x-ray because the arm needs to be manipulated to obtain the different views. If your child is in severe pain and /or there is an obvious deformity, your child will likely require a stronger pain medication than acetaminophen or ibuprofen. Please do not decline recommended pain medication for your child. You cannot feel the pain. I have seen parents decline medication with the reasoning that their child never complains. Well, this is the perfect time to give a pain reliever because it is clearly needed!

After the x-rays are performed your child's elbow will be placed in a splint and sling for immobilization. Many times, immobilizing the injured area provides a lot of pain relief because the arm is now supported.

The next steps depend on the x-ray results and where your child received medical care. If you brought your child to an urgent care center, the x-rays showed a nondisplaced fracture, and your child has adequate pain relief with immobilization and acetaminophen, your child may be referred to an outpatient orthopedist if it can be ensured that an appointment can be made for the following day.

However, your child will be sent to the emergency room for the following reasons: 1. Your child requires more pain management, 2. there is no available outpatient orthopedist for the nondisplaced fracture, 3. There is a displaced fracture.

If there is a clear deformity and your child cannot tolerate the x-rays, the elbow may be splinted for comfort and your child will be sent to the emergency room without getting any x-rays because it will be apparent that there is a displaced fracture. If the ends of the bone have a significant displacement, your child may need surgery. Most fractures heal without surgical intervention.

Fractures usually take approximately 6-8 weeks to heal. Your child should not participate in any gym or sports activities until cleared by the orthopedist.

Should Jared go?

No, Jared should not go to an urgent care center because he has a clear deformity. The humerus does not look like it is in a straight line. You do not need an x-ray to see that there is a fracture in this case. Jared should go directly to the emergency room.

Final Care Plan: Jared went directly to the emergency room. He reported having 9 out of 10 pain on the pain scale. He had significant tenderness over the elbow and was unable to move his arm, but his neurovascular exam was normal. He was given IV morphine prior to getting the x-rays. X-rays showed a displaced supracondylar fracture. The on-call orthopedist was consulted and placed Jared in a cast and sling. His parents were given instructions on fracture and splint home care, and he was discharged home with a scheduled follow-up appointment with the orthopedist.

Torus (Buckle/Incomplete) Fracture

Mary is a 6-year-old girl who has left ankle pain after slipping off the sidewalk curb and twisting her ankle yesterday. She only tolerated ice packs for a few minutes at a time. The ankle is swollen. No bruising is seen. She is not bearing weight on the left side. What is wrong with Mary's ankle?

Mary has a torus fracture of her left ankle. Torus fractures occur as a result of the bone getting compressed from pressure sustained from the injury. The compression creates a buckling of the bone that looks like a small bump on the shaft of the bone. Therefore, a torus fracture is also known as a buckle fracture. This can be seen on x-ray. Torus fractures occur most often on children's bones because their growth plates are still open and the bones are more flexible. It is also common to see a torus fracture of the lower ends of the forearm bones (e.g., radius, ulna) in the wrist region. This injury occurs after falling onto an outstretched hand.

Torus fractures should be splinted. Orthopedist follow-up can occur within the week as long as the injured limb is immobilized and pain management can be achieved with acetaminophen and ibuprofen.

Should Mary go?

Yes. Mary needs an exam of her entire upper extremity with a neurovascular examination of the area. Even if a fracture was not diagnosed, Mary should still be placed in a splint for comfort until the pain resolves.

Final Care Plan: Mary had moderate swelling and tenderness over one spot on the outer side of the left ankle. This is called point tenderness. Ankle x-rays showed a torus fracture of the lower end of the left fibula (i.e., the outer bone in the lower leg). Since Mary could not bear weight, she was placed in a splint and received crutches education.

*Please see the Crutches Instructions included in the Appendix.

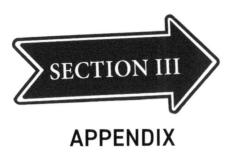

APPENDIX

Contusion Home Care Instructions for Bruises, Sprains, and Strains

- Acetaminophen (160mg/5ml): take as directed every 4 hours as needed for pain
- Children's Ibuprofen (100mg/5ml): take as directed every 6 hours as needed for pain
- Rest, ice, and elevate affected area (RICE). Apply ice or cold packs 15-20 minutes off and on 2-3 times per day as tolerated for the first 48 hours. You may shorten the time to 5-10 minutes off and on for younger children.
- No gym or sports for 5 days. If pain resolves, you can resume full activity.
- Follow up with an Orthopedist if there is no improvement in 3-5 days or complete resolution after 1 week of home care.

Splint Home Care Instructions

1. A splint is a supportive device used to immobilize an injured limb. Splinting in itself can provide pain relief. Splints can be formed and fitted for your child by using a material called fiberglass. The fiberglass is molded to fit your child and held in place by Ace bandages*.

2. Keep your child in the splint until pain resolves. You may remove the splint for icing, bathing, and sleeping.

3. Keep splint clean and dry. Do not apply ice while your child is wearing a splint. Use cold packs or remove the splint while icing. A wet splint does not feel nice.

4. If your child's arm is placed in a sling, make sure the sling is at a level where the forearm is parallel to the floor (the forearm makes a straight line across). Loosen or tighten the splint strap that goes around your child's neck as needed to accomplish this goal.

5. For finger splints: You may remove the splint to do range of motion exercises 2-3 times per day to prevent finger stiffness

6. For Ace bandage only splints: Keep on Ace wrap for compression.

7. You can use the time in the morning prior to putting the splint back on your child to test if the splint is no longer necessary. If your child has full range of motion and the pain has resolved, the splint is no longer needed.

*When using Ace wrap, do not stretch the bandage while wrapping. This will make the bandage too tight. You should be able to fit 2 fingers inside the bandage easily.

Fracture Home Care Instructions

- Acetaminophen (160mg/5ml): take as directed every 4 hours as needed for pain
- Children's Ibuprofen (100mg/5ml): take as directed every 6 hours as needed for pain.
- Do not remove cast or splint for bathing unless you were instructed to do so
- Rest, ice, and elevate the affected area (RICE).
- Apply ice packs for 15-20 minutes off and on 2-3 times per day as tolerated for the first 48 hours. You may shorten the time to 5-10 minutes off and on for younger children.
- You can elevate the limb by placing it on top of pillows.
- Keep splint or cast clean and dry. Protect from damage.
- There are waterproof cast and wound protectors available at your local pharmacy or store. If you cannot get one of these protectors, keep the splint/cast away from the water. (e.g., rest the splinted arm on the edge of the tub)
- Never put objects inside the cast to relieve itching.
- No weight bearing if so advised and use crutches as instructed.
- Watch for swelling, pain, burning, color change, numbness, or tingling. If these symptoms occur, elevate the extremity above the heart level for 30 minutes. If symptoms persist, go to the Emergency Department at once.
- Follow up with your Orthopedist for further care as advised.

Crutches Instructions

Crutches require balance and coordination. Your child should be able to bear weight on at least one foot. Most children cannot master the swinging motion of using traditional crutches until they are around age 7. If your child does not have good coordination and stumbles often, even if they are over the age of 7, you may want to avoid crutches. If crutches are provided during a medical evaluation, your child should be assessed to determine whether forearm crutches (crutches with forearm braces) may be an option for children who are younger and/or less coordinated if they are available. If forearm crutches are not available, a wheelchair may be recommended for your child. We will be discussing instructions for traditional crutches.

Check the Padding (if applicable):

If the crutches are new, the padding and grips should be adequate. If the crutches are used, check the padding on the armpit support, hand grip, and ferrules (the rubber cushions over the bases). If any of these parts are worn, they can be replaced by a medical supply store.

Set the Crutch Height:

Crutches are available in the following sizes: Child, Youth/Junior, Medium Adult, and Tall Adult. Most crutches require a minimum height of 4 feet 6 inches for use, but there are some available for children as short as 3 feet 8 inches.

Adjustable crutches have a height scale with 1-inch incre-ments. For aluminum crutches that have buttons for height adjustment, you can push the buttons and move the adjust-able legs up or down to the appropriate height. The handle height can also be adjusted by moving the handle screw to the appropriate notch. The handle screw is held in place by a hand-turned wing nut. Wooden crutches are a bit more tedious because they do not have a printed height scale on the side. Also, both the adjustable leg and handle are held in place with screws.

If you purchase your own crutches, you can deter-mine their correct height by setting them to your child's expected height. Have your child stand with the crutch-es. The crutches should be about 1 to 2 inches below your child's armpits (you should be able to fit 2 fingers between the armpit and the armpit pad). The handles should be at the height of your child's hips when held, with the elbows slightly bent.

*NOTE: Your child should rest his/her body weight on the crutch handles instead of the armpit cushions to avoid damaging the blood vessels and nerves in the armpits.

Different Crutch Maneuvers

How to Teach Your Child to Walk:

Your child should start in the standing position with the crutches approximately 4 to 6 inches out to the side and slightly in front of the feet. Next, your child should move both crutches forward a short distance (about half a stride). While using the handles for support, your child's body should swing forward and come down onto the good leg at the level or just past the crutches to complete the stride.

How to Teach Your Child to Get Up from a Chair:

Have your child place both crutches on the injured side (i.e., if the left leg was injured, both crutches should be held on the left side). Instruct your child to hold the chair arm-rest with one hand and the crutch handles with the other hand while pushing up.

How to Teach Your Child to Sit on a Chair:

Your child should back up to the seat of the chair. While keeping the injured extremity in front of the body, your child should hold both crutches on one hand and use the other hand to feel behind for the seat of the chair. Once the hand locates the seat, your child should sit down slowly. After sitting, the crutches should be leaned upside down in a nearby spot because crutches tend to fall over when they are leaned on their bases.

How to Teach Your Child to Use the Stairs:

GOING UPSTAIRS WITHOUT A HANDRAIL (OPTION 1):

Have your child stand close to the bottom step and place his/her weight on the crutches while bringing the foot on the good side onto the step. The injured leg and crutches can then be brought up onto the step. Repeat these motions for each step.

GOING UPSTAIRS USING A HANDRAIL (OPTION 2):
Have your child hold both crutches in one hand and hold the handrail with the other hand. Your child should place his or her weight on both hands to bring the foot on the good side onto the step. The injured leg and crutches can then be brought up onto the step. Repeat these motions for each step.

GOING DOWNSTAIRS:
Your child should go downstairs facing forward. First, have your child bend the knee on the good side to put the crutches on the lower step. Next, your child should place his/her weight on the crutch handles to hop down the step and land on the good foot. Repeat these motions for each step.

*Tip for School: Remember to ask your child's school to allow for dismissal from classes 5 minutes earlier and an elevator pass (if the school has an elevator) to allow time for travel between classes.

Medications That Should Be in Every Parent's Medicine Cabinet

The brand names are listed first. The generic names are in parentheses. The generic medications are equivalent to the brand name.

    a. Tylenol/FeverAll/Pediacare Fever Reducer and Pain Reliever (acetaminophen): take as directed every 4 hours as needed for fever or pain

    b. Motrin/Advil (ibuprofen): take as directed every 6 hours as needed for fever or pain

        i. AVOID IBUPROFEN ON AN EMPTY STOMACH OR IF COMPLAINING OF ABDOMINAL PAIN!

    c. Benadryl (diphenhydramine): take as directed every 6 hours as needed for itchiness or other allergy symptoms

        i. BENADRYL CAN CAUSE DROWSINESS!

    d. Claritin (loratadine) OR Zyrtec (cetirizine) OR Allegra (fexofenadine): take as directed 1-2 times per day as needed for allergy symptoms

        i. These allergies medications may cause drowsiness, but far less than diphenhydramine

        ii. These medications are all in the same family. Do NOT mix them together unless directed by your pediatrician or allergist. Pick ONE medication and use that one as needed.

e. Nasal saline spray: 1-2 sprays per nostril every 2-4 hours as needed to clear nasal passages

   i. You may use Nasal saline gel instead of the spray if desired, especially for dry nasal passages and after an epistaxis (nosebleed) episode

f. Cortizone-10 (Hydrocortisone 1% cream): Apply to affected areas 1-2 times per day as needed for itching

g. Children's Mylicon (simethicone): take as directed 3-4 times per day as needed for gassy symptoms

h. *Be careful to avoid combining medications with the same ingredients! ALWAYS CHECK THE LABEL!

   e.g. Many Cold & Flu medications contain acetaminophen. Do NOT mix these medications with plain acetaminophen!

Medications to AVOID

   a. Aspirin

   b. Ipecac

   c. Lomotil

   d. Pepto Bismol

*Medication Administration Tips

- For liquid/suspensions, use a medication syringe for accurate dosing. If your child is old enough to drink from a medicine cup, draw up the medication using the syringe and then place it in the medicine cup.

- You can ask your pharmacist if the medication can be flavored.

- Always ask your pharmacist whether a pill can be crushed or cut into smaller pieces.

- If your pill can be cut into smaller pieces, use a pill cutter. Pill cutters are available at your local pharmacy.

- You can try to disguise the medicine's taste by mixing it into fruit juice, applesauce, or pudding. This method can be used for liquids or crushed pills.

References

1. Atelectasis. Mayo Clinic. Mayo Foundation for Medical Education and Research (MFMER). 1998-2001. www.mayoclinic.org/diseases-conditions/atelectasis/symptoms-causes/syc-20369684.

2. Routine comprehensive care for children with sickle cell disease. Zora R Rogers MD. Literature review current through: Apr 2021. |This topic was last updated: Sep 26, 2020. www.uptodate.com/contents/routine-comprehensive-care-for-children-with-sickle-cell-disease?-search=sickle%20cell%20treatment&source=-search_result&selectedTitle=14~150&usage_type=default&display_rank=14.

3. Patel, Shilpa J. Patel and Teach, Stephen J. "Asthma." Pediatrics in Review November 2019, 40 (11) 549-567; DOI: https://doi.org/10.1542/pir.2018-0282.

4. COVID-19: Isolate If You Are Sick. www.cdc.gov/coronavirus/2019-ncov/if-you-are-sick/isolation.html. Page last updated Feb 18, 2021.

5. Nori, Kana. All you wanted to know about ambulation and how to make a video! SlideServe website. Uploaded Jul 19, 2014. www.slideserve.com/kana/

all-you-wanted-to-know-about-ambulation-and-how-to-make-a-video.

6. Crutches. The Royal Children's Hospital Melbourne. Last Reviewed. August 2020. www.rch.org.au/kidsinfo/fact_sheets/Crutches.

7. How to Use Crutches, Canes, and Walkers. American Academy of Orthopaedic Surgeons. Last reviewed Feb 2015. https://orthoinfo.aaos.org/en/recovery/how-to-use-crutches-canes-and-walkers.

Thank You

Thank you to the parents of my patients for trusting me to care for your children. Between your busy work schedules and lengthy commutes, I know that you do not want to unnecessarily pack up your children and schlep over to the doctor's office. As a pediatrician, I take the roles of healer and reassurer very seriously. It was your similar line of questioning that inspired me to write this book.

For a special BONUS for reading this book,

check out my FREE 3-part video series,

Do I Really Need to Take My Child to the Pediatrician Now?

Go to www.needtogopeds.com now!

About the Author

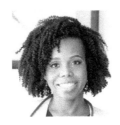

Dr. Sarah Irene Washington is a board-certified pediatrician, the chief medical director for Kiddo Care Pediatrics, and a pediatric urgent care physician. With more than a decade of experience in pediatrics, she has treated over forty thousand patients. At Kiddo Care Pediatrics, PLLC, Dr. Sarah Irene offers comprehensive medical care and provides honest, direct pediatric care that gives parents and children the personalized experience they deserve.

She obtained her Doctor of Medicine from the State University of New York (SUNY) Downstate Medical Center in Brooklyn, New York, and completed her pediatrics residency at Maria Fareri Children's Hospital at Westchester Medical Center in Valhalla, New York.

Dr. Sarah Irene is a native Brooklynite with roots in the South. She is a comedienne, classically trained pianist, author, caregiver of her mother, a sister, and aunt of two nieces. A world traveler, humanitarian, and philanthropist, she supports multiple organizations that sponsor and enrich children and underserved populations.

Learn more at drsarahirene.com

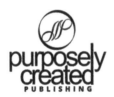

CREATING DISTINCTIVE BOOKS
WITH INTENTIONAL RESULTS

We're a collaborative group of creative masterminds
with a mission to produce high-quality books to position
you for monumental success in the marketplace.

Our professional team of writers, editors, designers,
and marketing strategists work closely together to ensure
that every detail of your book is a clear representation
of the message in your writing.

Want to know more?
Write to us at info@publishyourgift.com
or call (888) 949-6228

Discover great books, exclusive offers, and more at
www.PublishYourGift.com

Connect with us on social media

@publishyourgift